ACUPRESSURE

(Holistic Approach to Make Life Better)

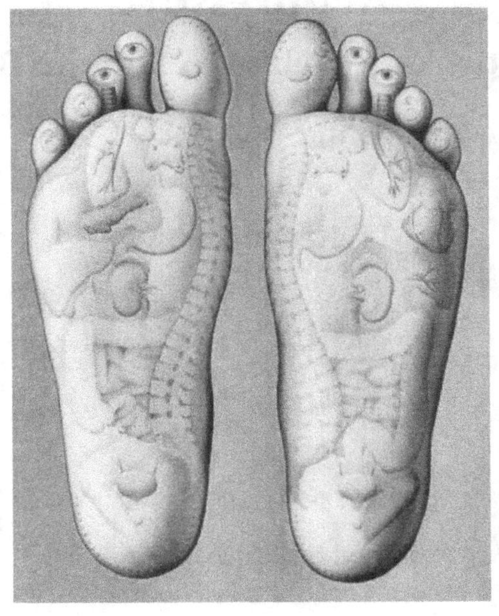

Dr. Kamaljit Singh

RIGI PUBLICATION

All right reserved

No part of this book may be reproduced in any form, by Photostat, Microfilm, xerography, or any other means or incorporated into any information retrieval system, Electronic or Mechanical, Without the Written Permission of the copyright owner.

Acupressure
(Holistic Approach to Make Life Better)

BY

Dr. Kamaljit Singh

Copyright © Dr. Kamaljit Singh 2022

Originally published in India

ISBN: 978-93-91041-33-5

Published by RIGI PUBLICATION

777, Street no.9, Krishna Nagar

Khanna-141401 (Punjab), India

Website: www.rigipublication.com

Email: info@rigipublication.com

Phone: +91-9357710014, +91-9465468291

DEDICATION

This book is dedicated to my mother. My mother **Late Smt. Surinder Kaur** was a woman like no other. She gave me life, nurtured me, taught me, dressed me, fought for me, shouted at me, kissed me, but most importantly she loved me unconditionally. There are no enough words to describe just how important my Mother is to me and what a powerful influence she continued to be.

I awake each morning to start a new day But the pain of losing you never goes away I go about the things I have to do
And as the hours pass I think again of you I want to call you and just hear your voice Then I remember that I have no choice
For you are not there and how my heart cries Just to see you again to tell you goodbye To say Maa I love you and I always will
And hope that much of you, in me you've instilled The day that you left I just didn't know
That you were going where I couldn't go And now all my memories of you are so dear
But gosh, how I miss you and wish you were here Who now can hear me when I need to cry?
It is so hard to tell you "Mom goodbye"
Someday I know all will be well
and I'll see you again with stories to tell
Of how you were missed and how we have grown and how good it is to finally be home
Until then my memories of you I'll keep near and I'll pass them on to those who are dear.

In the sweet memory of her. This book titled **"Neuro Acupressure - Holistic Approach for Healthy Livings"** is dedicated to her.

Dr. Kamaljit Singh

PREFACE

The menace of spurious drugs, the dangerous side effects of numerous medicines, the alarming figures of various diseases and above all costly medical treatment has remained a matter of serious concern for a majority of our people. I had an abiding interest in Health Science since my School time. My curiosity was amply rewarded in 1993 when I got an opportunity to study Health Science (Alternative Medicines) from International Institute of Alternative Medicines. I have developed a strong inclination for a Holistic Approach to Healthy Livings which could extend the much needed cure to patients promptly, effectively and at a nominal cost. I came to know that Acupressure Therapy was put to test in USA and found very useful. I went deep into it and found its roots in India as 5000 years ago.

Acupressure is only an offspring of Nature's own science installed in our body and given as a great boon to mankind. Acupressure therapy was being followed in different forms in different countries and even the Red Indians in 16th century cured disease by pressing different points on the patient's soles. Dr. William Fitzgerald and others of USA have carried out research on the same and have brought this science to light in the 20th century.

This therapy is capable of solving the present world health problems and bestowing good health on all in just couple of years.

From the view point of health the world could be divided into:

1. (About 60%) – those people (including those to be born) who are healthy but liable to catch diseases. With the regular Acupressure treatment their illness can be prevented.
2. (About 25%) – those people who are suffering at present but can be cured with minimum cost with the help of this science and prevented from falling ill again.
3. (About 15%) – who require medical help, medicine and or surgery. There are enough practitioners and hospitals in the world that can take care of these people. Afterwards they can also be prevented from falling ill, with the use of acupressure therapy.

Thus with proper propagation and teaching of this science, most of the health problems of the world can be solved. This can be done easily a mentioned below;

a. The therapy should be learnt by the teachers of high schools and professors at the college level and taught as a voluntary subject. These students, in turn, will propagate this therapy not only in their homes but also in community around and during their vacations.
b. Retired teachers, professors, government servants and other educated people can learn it and conduct classes to teach it to others.
c. The social media can greatly assist by regularly publishing articles on various aspects of this therapy and the experiences of their readers/viewers.
d. Philanthropists and charitable organizations, religious minded people and religious institutions can adopt this as a "God Given Therapy" and work for its propagation.

The huge amount which is being spent on health problems can better be diverted towards better hygiene, better and cheaper supply of nutritious food to the people and thus create a good will cycle to bring health, wealth and happiness to all.

The World Health Organization (W.H.O) is now giving attention to this therapy. The West has accepted acupuncture. Very soon the World will accept this Health Science which is the mother of Acupuncture, Shiatsu, Sujok or pointed pressure therapy.

We shall always be grateful to those unknown Rishis or sages who discovered the reflex points installed in our palms and soles to be pressed for treatment under this therapy and made us aware of these points. We are also grateful to all those who have preserved this science through and centuries and also those who helped to encourage this science.

Dr. Kamaljit Singh
Author - (Holistic Approach for Healthy Livings)

FOREWARD

The book written by Dr. Kamaljit Singh on Neuro Acupressure Therapy (Foot and Hand Reflexology), making available simple directions for using the Neuro Acupressure therapy to preserve one's good health and to cure common to chronic ailments.

The human body is a perfect machine which can regulate itself, provided the natural rules of food, work and rest are observed. When we transgress natural rules, we create toxins in the body, which the body attempts to get rid of. This attempt is considered as disease and is given different names according to different symptoms. If the transgression of rules is set right by natural methods available to every human being, complete cure is possible without any other aid. This is Holistic Approach for Healthy Livings to Make Life Better which includes the following methods:

- Fasting as long as necessary and then dieting properly, using colon detox Tea, Far Infra- Red Sauna System, Ultra Sonic/Ion Bubble Bath, Foot Detox Spa etc.

- Using wheat grass juice along with raw diet.

- Living only on fresh and raw vegetables, to be taken regularly in a proper manner. Using Bio Magnets to cure ailments as prescribed in this book.

- Adopting Neuro Acupressure Therapy which is described in this hand book in simple language with clear instructions.

- Doing regular pranayama and yoga asana

- Every person can use any one or more of these methods according to his conviction and convenience. What is required is "faith in the therapy/treatment adopted."

- Sincere thanks to my wife **Mrs. Balwinder Kaur** and son **Harsimranjit Singh** for their support to write this book.

- My great gratitude to respected **Sardar Sukhdev Singh** (Lecturer Physics), who has blessed me with his guidance and encouraged me to write this book so that who so ever is interested in Holistic approach for healthy livings can take advantages of this book.

Dr. Kamaljit Singh

Managing Director/Chief Consultant

Dr. Kamal Bio Magnetic Holistic Health Centre Bangkok (Thailand)

FOREWARD

Er. Bikramjit Singh Khalsa
Member

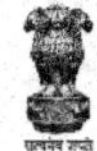

Punjab Public Service Commission
Patiala- 147 001
Ph. : 0175-5014814 (Off.)
0175-5014831 (Fax)

Dated......................

It's my pleasure and privilege and I feel honored to contribute my views about Dr. Kamaljit Singh and the book "Acupressure" (Holistic Approach to Make Life Better).

Dr. Kamaljit Singh is our family friend (Like a brother), very humble personality. We have visited his Dr. Kamal Bio Magnetic Wellness Centre Bangkok couple of times and experienced his vast knowledge about Alternative therapies and his Centre was well equipped with the Sophisticated Health Care Therapies such as Ozone Bath, Far Infra -Red Sauna System, Foot Detox, Quantum Resonance Magnetic Health Analyzer, Acupressure and Magnetic healing devices etc.

Now about this Book it's a fully illustrated and comprehensive reference guide to acupressure

· Provides acupressure treatments tailored for a wide variety of health disorders, including back pain, heart and circulatory problems, and even the common to chronic ailments.

· Contains step-by-step instructions illustrated for self-treatment or treatment of others

Acupressure confers a holistic health benefit that prevents disorder from arising by harmonizing and balancing the body's energies. It is particularly suited to self-treatment, the treatment of others, and especially the treatment of children. Along with an introduction to the origins and principles of Alternative Medicines, This hand held Acupressure book provides the most important basic techniques as well as step-by-step instructions of the practical and specific information needed to put the healing techniques of acupressure at your fingertips.

I convey my best wishes to Dr. Kamaljit Singh for his services to the mankind in order to buildup happier and healthier nation with less sufferings.

Ex MLA

RAJIV GANDHI NATIONAL UNIVERSITY OF LAW, PUNJAB
(Established under Punjab Act No. 12 of 2006)
(Accredited with 'A' Grade by NAAC)

Dr. Jasleen Kewlani
ASSISTANT PROFESSOR OF SOCIOLOGY
Editor, RGNUL Social Science Review (RSSR)
B.A. (Vocational with Functional Eng.),
M.A. (Sociology), UGC (NET), Ph.D.,
UGC Research Awardee (Post Doc),

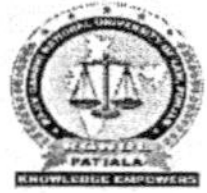

Telephone : +91-175-2391376 (O)
Mobile : +91-9501225855 (M)
E-mail : jasleenkewlani@gmail.com
rgnulrjs@rgnul.ac.in
jasleen@rgnul.ac.in

Foreword

I feel honoured, since I am contributing a few words in grace of a very good human being and a very skilled and professionally efficient doctor. Dr. Kamaljit Singh has established is name worldwide in the field of Bio Magnetic Holistic Health and has made many people live a disease free and pain free life with his treatment. I congratulate him for his present venture, this book entitled, "Acupressure (Holistic Approach to Make Life Better".

Dr. Kamaljit's name has been well recognised in association with his service to the Armed forces and Indian Navy. His presence in the Indian Cricket team for uncountable years has also made him leave an unforgettable mark on the team members, their health and their success too. After serving the prominent national groups of professionals, Dr. Kamaljit has dedicated his commitment to the field of natural care and therapeutic treatment of the persons in sufferings.

When people like him write, they speak reality of life along with many facts and solutions to innumerable problems. This book authored by Dr. Kamaljit also opens up many unfolded aspects of knowledge regarding Neuro Acupressure and human anatomy. The contents of this book guide the readers about the repairing of the worn out and damaged body organs and also for generating strength from within one's own life and living routines.

I very humbly once again congratulate Dr. Kamaljit and all the team members associated with him in all his endeavours for the publication of this book. I am sure that this book shall benefit uncountable people and shall bring them out of their pains and medical ailments. I recommend this boon strongly and also ask Dr. Kamaljit to keep writing for the general good of the common people.

Best Wishes,

Dr. Jasleen Kewlani Rambani
University Grants Commission Research Awardee (Post Doc)
&
Assistant Professor of Sociology, RGNUL
Chief Editor, RGNUL Social Sciences Review (RSSR)
Rajiv Gandhi National University of Law, Patiala, Punjab
Contact No. 09501225855

Sidhuwal, Bhadson Road, Patiala - 147 006 (Punjab), INDIA. Tel.: +91-175-2391200 Fax: +91-175-2391690
E-mail: info@rgnul.ac.in website: www.rgnul.ac.in

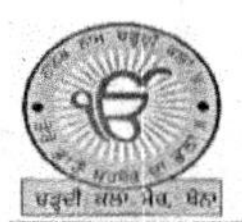

ਚੜ੍ਹਦੀ ਕਲਾ ਮੰਚ, ਖੰਨਾ (ਪੰਜਾਬ)

ਮੋਬਾਇਲ 94633-04544

ਕ੍ਰਮ ਅੰਕ...1.......   ਮਿਤੀ 29.7.2022

Few Words

    I write my views about the book in your hand named Accupressure, before that, I want to write few words about Dr. Kamaljit singh, an international fame personality. He is one in the list of best students of my teaching carrier. After schooling he joined Indian Navy and served for 15 years. During his service period he got diploma in Magnetic Therapy. After retiring from Indian Navy, he captured huge knowledge of Anatomy of Human body and adopted the profession of a doctor after getting in alternative medicine. Serving humanity by AM (alternative medicine) is not his profession but passion. He not only has given his medical services in Oman, Singapore Malasia but run successfully Holistic Health centre at Bangkok (Thiland) nearly 15 years. Now on my advice he has started his clinic in Khanna (Pb) his native land. I am realy proud of him.

    Let us Now talk about his first Book Accupressure It is complete book in all respects. In the bigining he wrote about Human Anatomy and then ethics of a practitioner. There is complete knowlegde of Nerve Accupressure that is reflex points in hands, feet and other parts of body. According to book accupressure therapy not only diagonsis the root cause of a decease but finds its intensity, cures and prevent our body from serious deceases. I am confident that his book is not benificial for therapist only but for a common person for their body fitness to make life better.

Sukhdev Singh
(Retd. Lecturer Physics)
Founder
Charhdi Kala Manch,
Khanna (Pb)

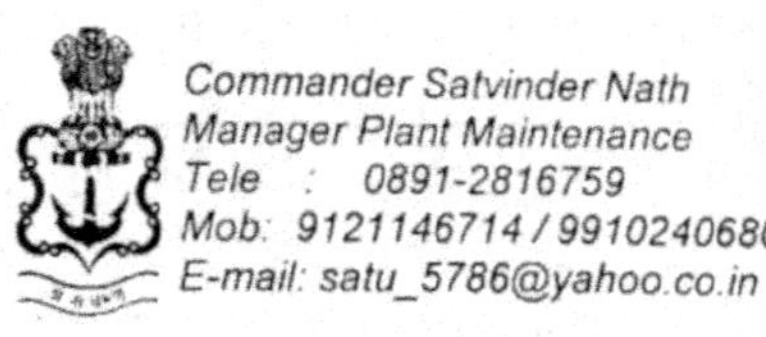
Commander Satvinder Nath
Manager Plant Maintenance
Tele   :   0891-2816759
Mob: 9121146714 / 9910240680
E-mail: satu_5786@yahoo.co.in

Naval Dockyard
C/o Fleet Mail Office
Visakhapatnam - 530 014

It gives me immense pleasure to know that Dr. Kamaljit Singh MD/Chief Consultant, Bio Magnetic Holistic Health Centre has come up with more appropriate book on the subject of Neuro Acupressure Therapy.

After putting of successful and challenging two decades tenure in Armed Forces/ Indian Navy service Dr. Kamaljit Singh has explored his passion for health science and achieved great heights in the field of natural cure. He further went on to explore his writing skills and come up with a book on Neuro Acupressure – To Make Life Better.

The book clearly shows the amount of research being carried out by Dr. Kamaljit Singh in bringing out all aspects of Neuro Acupressure in this master piece. It's an eye opening book which gives clear understanding of acupressure as a "God Given Therapy" to bring good health, wealth and happiness to all. Additionally the book explains full human anatomy, its natural way of repairing of worn out & damaged organs and generating strength and vigour.

This book is a must read for better understanding of human body and its natural method of healing itself. I would like to complement Dr. Kamaljeet Singh for touching all aspects of Neuro Acupressure therapy and enlighten everyone on this natural healing technique.

My best wishes.

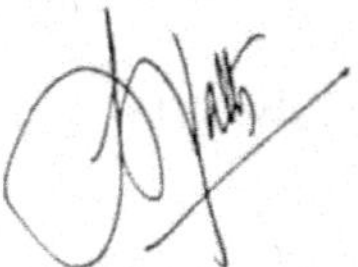

TABLE OF CONTENTS

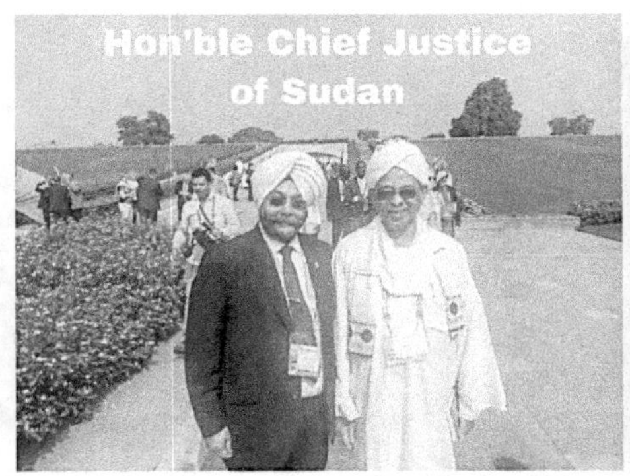

Hon'ble Chief Justice
of Sudan

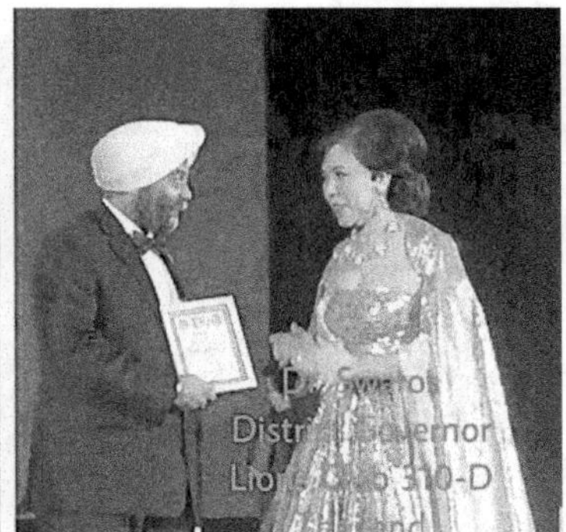

District Governor
Lions Club 310-D

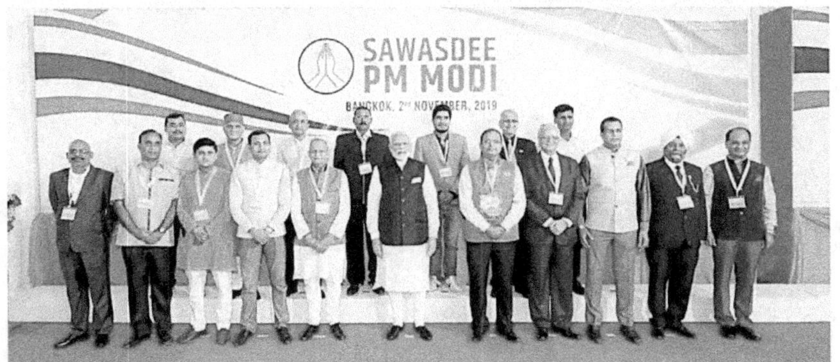

SAWASDEE
PM MODI
BANGKOK, 2nd NOVEMBER, 2019

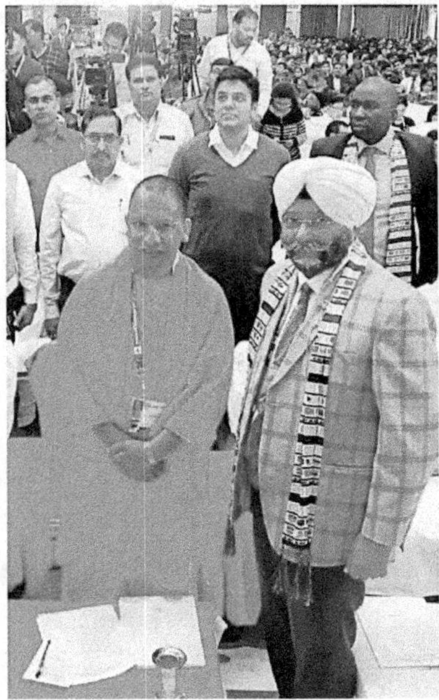

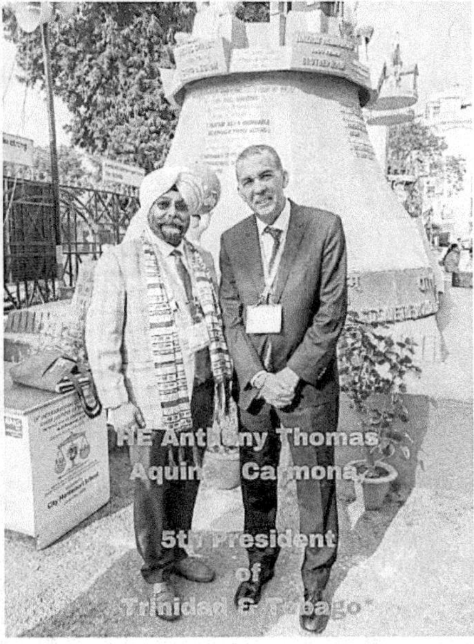

HE Anthony Thomas
Aquinas Carmona
5th President
of
Trinidad & Tobago

1. HUMAN BODY – AN INTRODUCTION

Seven wonders are believed to be there in the world. But if there is something which is most wonderful and amazing, it is our body which is a living machine made up of several parts. There are several organs and sub organs in our body just as there are several big and small components in a machine. It is however a natural machine which differs a lot from an artificial or manmade machine. Our body not only functions like a machine but also generates energy and vigor in itself. It is such a machine which requires no operator. This machine itself repairs the worn out and damaged organs, besides accomplishing many simple and complex tasks, generating strength and vigor. Waste matters are also thrown out of the body due to this mechanism. Body keeps growing gradually in size. It possesses an amazing power of performing various functions by responding to external influences. This is why it has been called a high quality remarkable machine.

Different organs of the body are outwardly visible, but there are some organs which are inside the body. We cannot see them directly but keep functioning all the time.

1.01. **Cells**: Just like other creatures, human body is also formed by a group of cells. Each cell is structural and functional unit of human body.

HUMAN CELLS

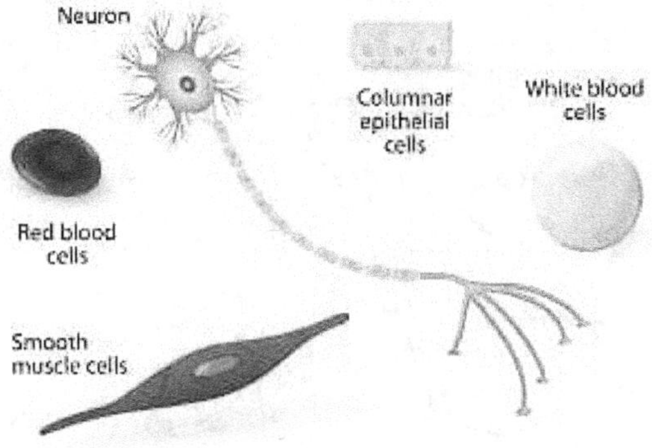

1.02. **Tissues**: When many cells having similar structure perform one function then they are collectively referred to as "Tissues"

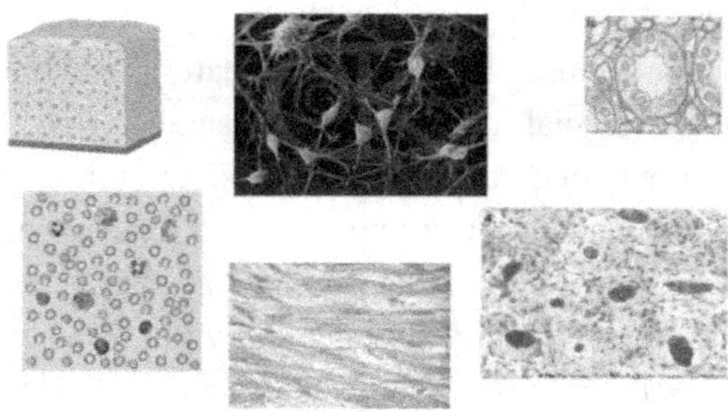

1.03. **Organs**: Those parts of the body which perform specific functions and which are formed by several tissues together are called organs.

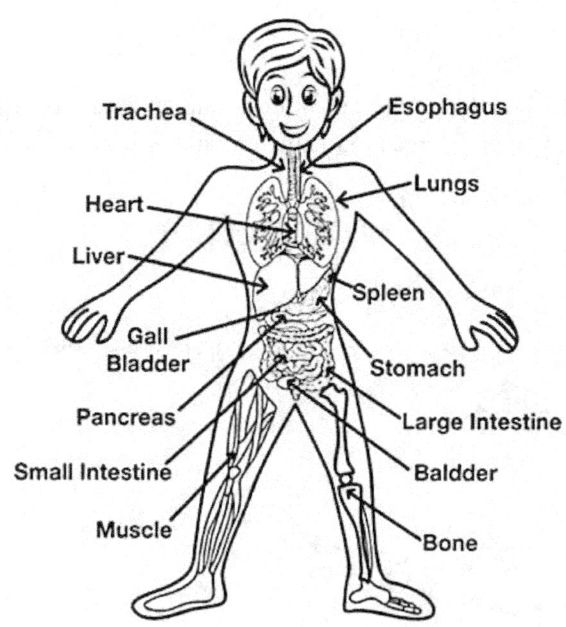

1.04. **System:** When several organs perform one particular function then it is termed as system.

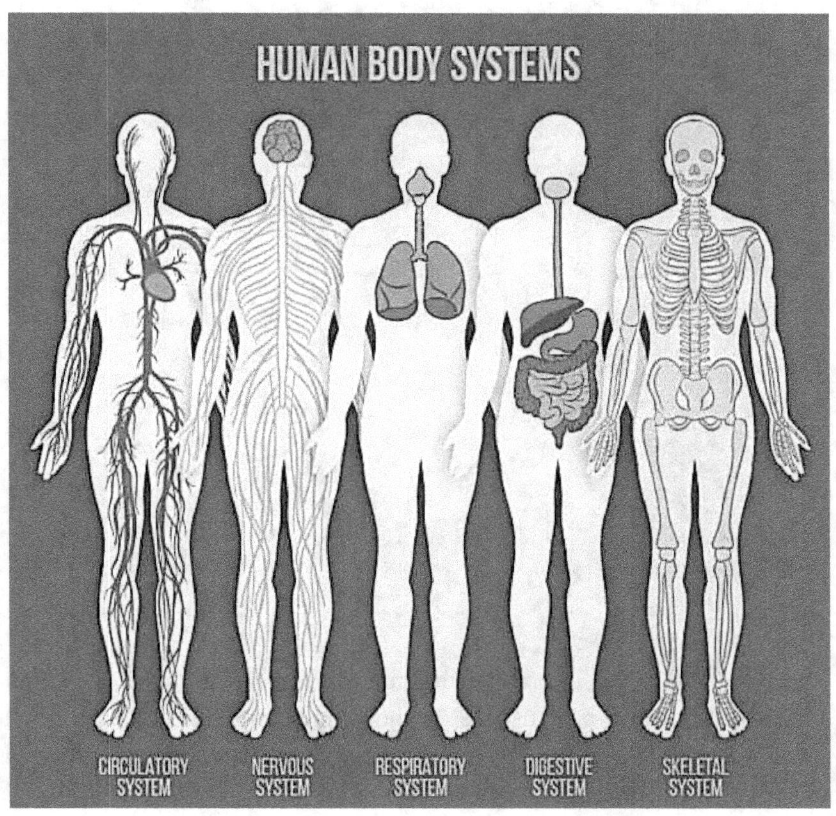

1.05. **Skeleton System:** Skeleton supports the body just as the support of iron or concrete pillar is needed for constructing a mansion. There can be no shape or form of body without bones. By seeing the ingenuity of nature in the making of bones, one wonder as to how much a tiny framework can be so strong. The weight of bones is less from the point of view of firmness and strength. One bone is five times as strong as Sheeshum, the hardest wood. A bone of one square inch has the capacity to bear a load of nearly 2 tons. Calcium salts, which we get from our meals, impart firmness, stiffness and strength to bones.

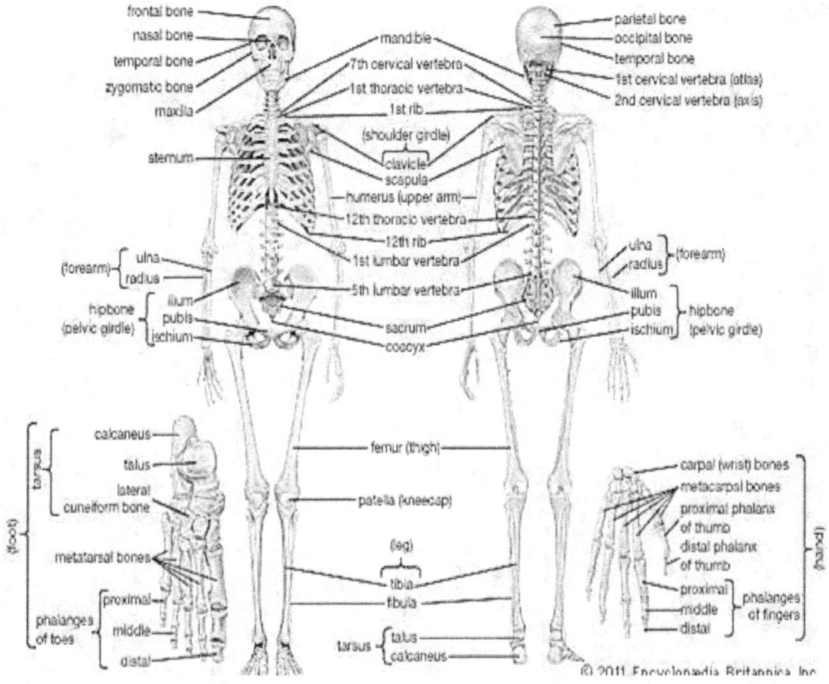

There are 270 bones in body at the time of birth which reduces to 206. Some bones join to become one. For example there are 33 bones in the spine. Later on however 5 bones combine to form with sacrum while 4 bones combine to form coccyx.

There is no friction among bones and they perform all the actions without making sounds as there is flow of synovial liquid in joint capsule.

There are 78% solid matters (34% organic solid, 44% inorganic matters) and 22% water in our bones.

Skeleton acts like a framework and supports delicate tissues. It has the capacity to make free movements with the help of muscles. It protects delicate organs within body. Body corpuscles are produced in the spongy area of the long bones, the ribs and vertebrae.

1.06.   Muscular System: There are several delicate organs inside the framework of bones which remain attached to these bones with the help of fibrous tissues. There are many types of glands which do the vital job of sustaining the body. There are muscles for covering the bones and protecting glands and delicate organs and imparting physique. Above these muscles is fat and above these is skin which is visible on the surface. Muscles are there everywhere in the body in varying quantities. Muscles facilitate all the actions in the body. Moving, sitting, standing, opening mouth, speaking, winking, beating of heart and breathing are some of the actions which are conducted by muscles. Muscles attached to skeleton are made up of several tiny pieces. Muscles remain linked with each other through fibers tissues. The peculiar characteristic of muscle is that it can contract and become fatter and smaller and regains its previous position.

Muscles contain 75% water and 25% protein. They also contain potassium and Sulphur in small quantity. On being squeezed, a juice trickles from fresh meat, which clots after sometime. Juice contained in the muscles clots after death. Consequently muscles in body become stiff. It happens due to clotting of protein. Muscles become devoid of capacity to contract and expand after death.

There are two types of movements in the body: Voluntary and involuntary.

Voluntary Controlled action taking place according to our will e.g. moving, speaking, chewing food etc. These are called voluntary actions.

Involuntary actions are ones which are not in our control e.g. beating of heart. We cannot prevent it from beating.

Our body houses more than 600 muscles which have been different names based on their size, length and position. Muscles are linked to brain through well-defined system. Our organs are active but they do not act on their own. It is the function of the muscles to produce actions in them. Muscles are of three types:

1.06.01.Voluntary Muscles: Movements occur because of these muscles. We can contract or expand these muscles as per our will. Such types of muscles are found on the upper layer of the body. This is why they are referred to as skeletal muscles; also since they act according to our will, they are also called controlled muscles.

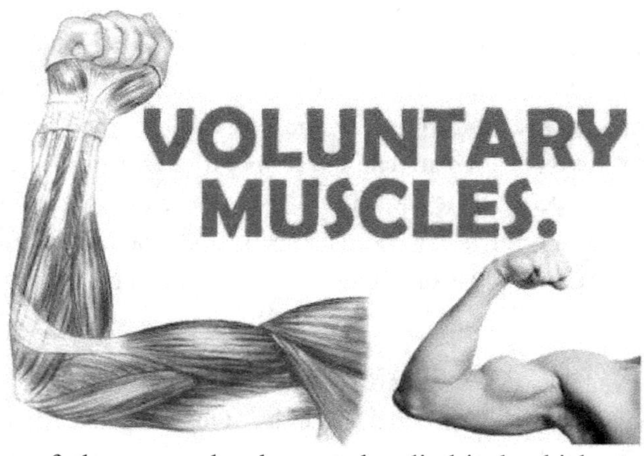

The fibers of these muscles long and cylindrical which appear like distinct striations. These muscles are responsible for giving shape to the body and storing energy.

1.06.02. Involuntary Muscles: These muscles are found in internal organs and therefore they are so called visceral muscles, e.g. stomach, blood vessels etc. These muscles receive their signals from a different network of nerves, the autonomic system. These muscles function automatically and we usually are not even aware of their action. We cannot expand or contact them as per our will. These muscles are not connected to any bone. They are white in color as they devoid of blood cells.

1.06.03. Cardiac Muscles: Though the structure of cardiac muscles is similar to that of voluntary muscles, they are in fact involuntary muscles, as their action is not dependent on our will. They keep expanding and contracting on their own. Stripes are found on cardiac muscle despite their belonging to the category of involuntary muscles. But their strips are not as conspicuous as those of voluntary muscles.

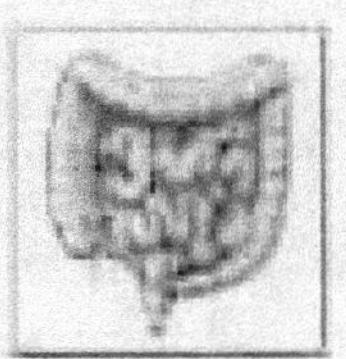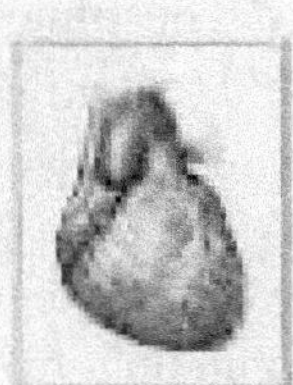

1.06.04. Importance of Muscles: Muscles are store house of physical strength; we cannot see muscles as the body is enveloped by skin. Muscles offer protection to bones by covering them and make the body strong and well built. It is only due to muscles that there is movement in bones and the body performs various functions. Energy and heat is generated in muscles due to chemical process in muscles which imparts vigor and vibrancy to the body enabling it to carry out various functions. Energy enhances the capacity of muscles to function and heat maintains body temperature.

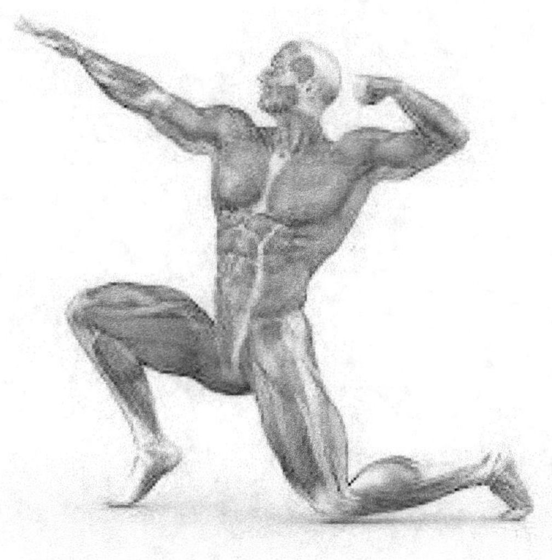

1.07. Circulatory System: The Supply of nutrients as well as oxygen in adequate quantity to each and every tissue and organ is required to enable them to carry out their respective functions. Besides, managing the breakdowns resulting from various bodily functions is also a must. Both these functions are carried out in body of the humans by blood. Normally blood constitutes 5% of the weight of the body. There are approximately 70,000 miles of blood vessels in the body. Circulation of blood takes place through arteries, veins and capillaries.

1.07.01. Artery: Pure blood flows in it. The walls of vessels are flexible and thick. Originating from the heart is spread across the body and carries blood to it.

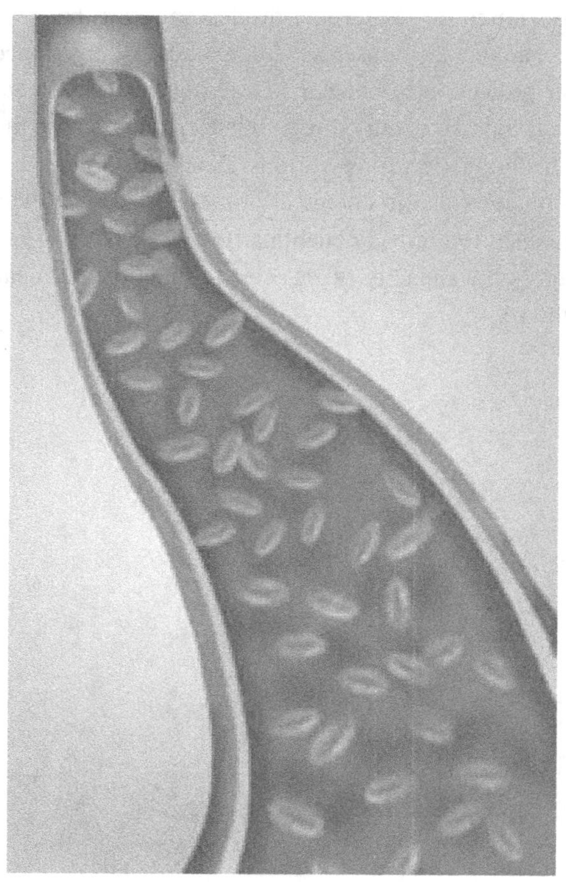

1.07.02. Veins: Impure blood flows in it. The walls of the vessels are thin and weak.

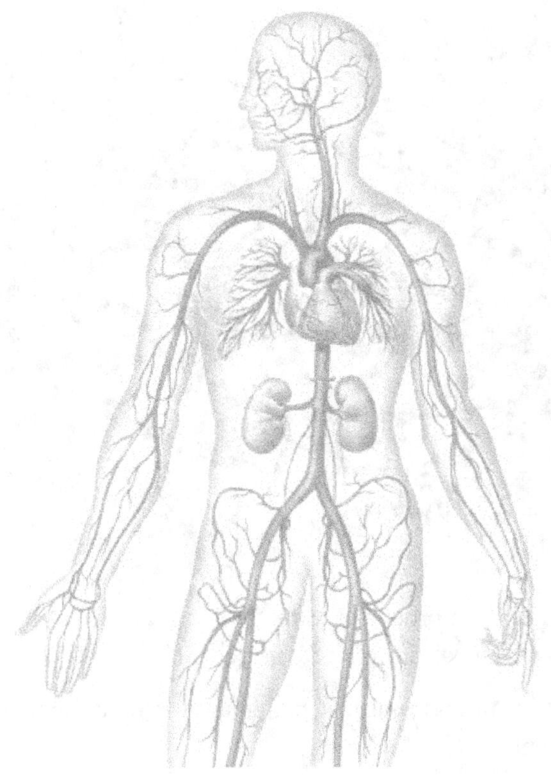

1.07.03. Capillaries: Spread throughout the body like a net, capillaries are thinner than hair. They are sandwiched between arteries and veins like a junction.

1.08. Blood:

A. Cells 45% of blood volume
Red Blood Corpuscles (RBC)
White Blood Corpuscles (WBC)
Platelets & Thrombocytes (TC)

B. Plasma 55% (Water 90% Solids 10%)

1.08.01. Functions of Blood Circulation:

-Carrying oxygen to the body- It gets fresh oxygen from the lungs and supplies it to all parts of the body.

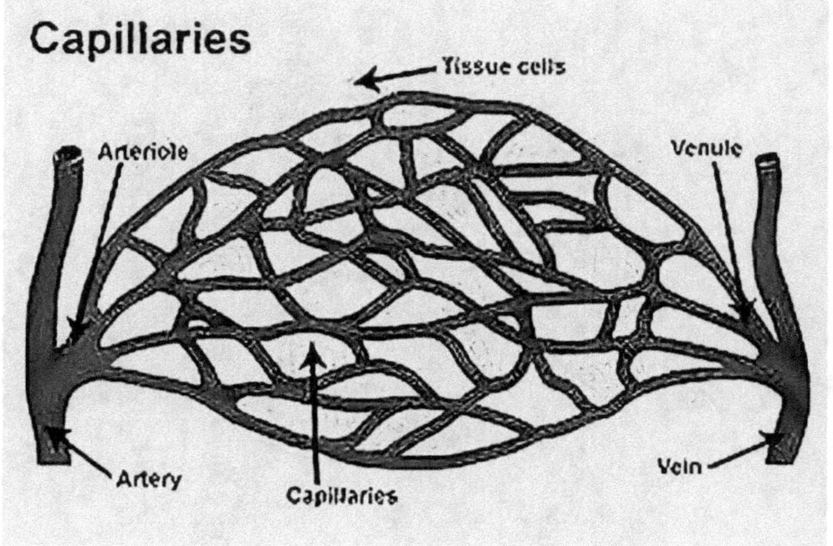

-It carries carbon dioxide produced in the body as a result of performing various activities to lungs from where it is ejected.

-With the help of skin and lungs, it maintains the body temperature at 98.4 degree Fahrenheit.

-It carries various types of waste matter produced in the body tissue to excretory organs and facilitates their expulsion out of the body.

-It carries hormones produced by endocrine glands to vital organs.

-Protects the body by destroying disease causing organisms

-Nurtures all the organs of the body.

-Provides humidity to the body.

1.09. Heart: The heart is a muscular organ about the size of two clenched fists. It consists of a double pump located a little to the left of the middle of chest behind the breast bone. It lies enclosed in a sac called pericardium and is surrounded by the lungs.

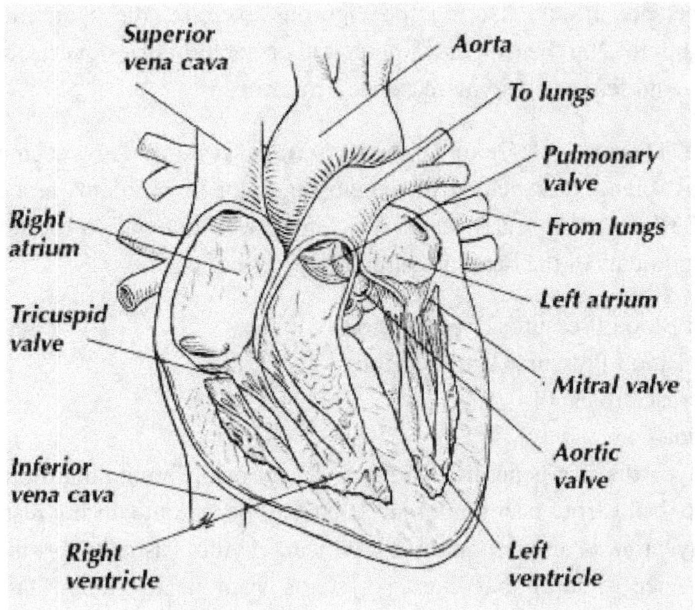

After a few days following conception until death, the heart continues to beat, never stopping to rest except for a fraction of second between beats. The heart alternatively contracts to empty and relaxes to fill and this action is called heartbeat. The interior of the heart contains four main chambers, the atria (right and left) and the ventricles (right and left). The atria are upper chambers, which receive blood into circulation. The ventricles are discharging chambers which pump blood from the heart into circulation. The ventricles meet at the bottom of the heart to form a pointed base which points towards the left side of the chest. The blood in the heart keeps flowing in the right direction by a system of valves. These four valves open and close automatically to let blood pass through and prevent it from flowing backwards.

Heart is made up of a muscle called cardiac muscle which constricts and relaxes about 70-80 minute. As the cardiac muscle contracts, it pushes the blood through the chambers into the vessels. The nervous system regulates the speed at which the muscle contracts. The heart rate is fastest in infancy, about 120 beats per minute. As the child grows the heart rate slows. By the age of 18, the heart rate has stabilized to about

70 beats per minute. During the vigorous exercise, the heart rate can reach up to 200 beats per minute. Other factors like fever, anemia, anxiety and fear can also increase the heart rate.

1.09.01. Diseases of Heart and circulatory system: Advancement in medical science has helped in diagnosing a lot of problems associated with the heart at an early stage. Two most well-known (to the popular mind) ailments of the heart are circulatory system is;

- High Blood Pressure (Hypertension)
- Low Blood Pressure (Hypotension)
- Atherosclerosis
- Angina
- Tachycardia is a general term for a variety of different conditions that cause the heart to beat more than 100 times per minute during rest.
- Bradycardia is an abnormally s36w heart rhythm (usually less than 60 beats per minute) that causes systems such as dizziness, fainting, extreme tiredness and shortness of breath.
- Coronary thrombosis is the development of a blood clot in one of the arteries supplying blood to the heart, as a result of which the blood circulation to that area of heart muscle stops. This is also called as myocardial infraction or heart attack.
- Heart failure is a condition that can result from any structural or functional cardiac disorder that impairs the ability of the heart to fill with the pump a sufficient amount of blood throughout the body.
- Heart block
- Valvular heart disease is abnormality of one or more of heart's four valves.
- Cardiac enlargement is increase in the size of the heart.
- Varicose veins are enlarged veins close to skin surface, most commonly affected are those in the legs and feet.
- Pericardial effusion is presence of abnormal amount of fluid in pericardial space.
- Congenial heart disease the general name for over forty types of birth defects of the heart and blood vessels is present in about six babies out of every thousand live births.

- Despite the fact that new diagnostic techniques, drugs and interventions are continually being introduced in medical science, there is a constant rise in the number of patients suffering from heart diseases. Unhealthy lifestyle lack of proper exercise, irregular eating habits, smoking, excessive alcohol consumption, mental stress, over work, lack of proper sleep are all conditions which favor the development of heart diseases.

1.09.02. Blood Pressure:

- Blood pressure is very variable. It varies from person to person and even in different parts of the body. For the sake of convenience, doctors normally measure it in one of the large arteries of an arm. Blood pressure is the force of blood against the walls of arteries. Blood pressure is recorded as two numbers—the systolic pressure (as the heart beats) over the diastolic pressure (as the heart relaxes between beats). The measurement is written one above or before the other, with the systolic number on top and the diastolic number on the bottom. For example, a blood pressure measurement of 120/80 mmHg (millimeters of mercury) is expressed verbally as "120 over 80."

- Normal blood pressure is less than 120 mmHg systolic and less than 80 mmHg diastolic.

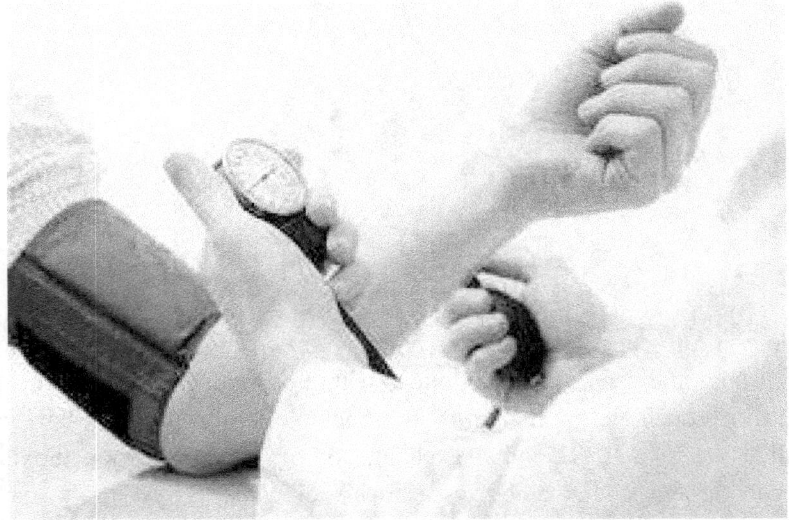

Age	Systolic	Diastolic
20	118	78
25	120	80
30	122	82
35	124	84
40	127	86
45	130	88
50	133	90
55	138	92
60	143	94
65	148	96

1.10   Respiratory System: We breathe in order to supply the body with the oxygen essential for energy production, and to get rid of carbon dioxide, which is a waste product of energy production. At the Centre of respiratory system are the lungs, where breathed in oxygen is exchanged for carbon dioxide from the blood. The channel along which air is breathed in and out of lungs consists primarily of the nose, throat and trachea.

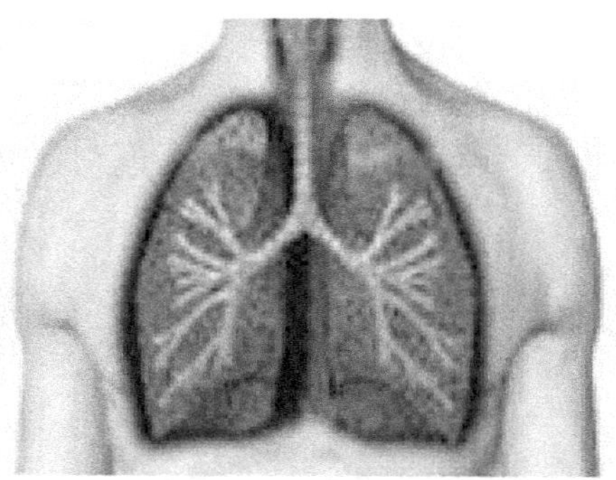

-Deep in the chest, the trachea divides into two main bronchi, one for each lung and each bronchus divides within each lung into increasingly smaller bronchioles, at the tip of all bronchioles are balloon like cavities called the alveoli. The vital exchange of oxygen for carbon dioxide occurs through minute blood vessels in alveoli walls.

-The human respiratory system is a very flexible one. Whereas at rest the lungs shift 5-8 liters of air a minute they can increase 20-30 fold to up to about 200 liters a minute.

Common disorders of the lungs are: asthma, bronchitis, pneumonia, pleurisy, cough, allergies etc.

1.10.01.Asthma: It is a disease of the respiratory system in which the airways constrict, became inflamed and are lined with excessive amount of mucous, often in response to one or more triggers such as exposure to an environmental stimulant (allergen), cold, air, exercise, cigarette smoke or emotional stress. This airway narrowing causes symptoms such as wheezing, shortness of breath, chest congestion and cough.

These remarks apply to bronchial asthma usually referred to simply asthma. However, there is one other form of asthma called cardiac asthma which usually occurs at night in middle age or elderly people. It is due to left heart failure. The exact cause of asthma is not completely known.

-The immune system over reacts to triggers and cause the airways to become inflamed and tight. Asthma is characterized by periodic flare ups. Between flare ups, many people return to normal breathing. Over years this pattern can continue without the person getting dramatically worse.

-Asthma can be diagnosed by pulmonary function tests. However there is no effective cure for asthma. With medicines, only the acute phase can be relieved. This however does not prevent future attacks; some people are misguided by the quacks and consume a dubious medicine which contains steroids. This may bring immediate relief but later on they have a very harmful effect on the body. Steroids have been found in many local medicines when tested in the laboratory.

Prevention:
- The best way to prevent asthma is to identify and avoid indoor and outdoor allergy and irritants.
- Several studies shown that Yoga to be a powerful adjunct therapy to reduce the frequency and intensity of asthma attacks as well as

decrease medication use. Consistent practice of Yoga postures of breathing techniques increase the air flow of lungs, air capacity, stamina and efficiency. Back-bending exercises open the chest improving both lungs and heart functioning. Breathing techniques cultivates the ability to maintain a relaxed and controlled breath that can prevent or reduce asthmatic attacks. To help strengthen the lungs and reduce mucous congestion use "Kapalbhati" breathing techniques, practicing it very slowly and gently in short durations.

- Monitor your breathing; learn to recognize the warning signs of impending attack such as slight coughing or shortness of breath. The lung function may decrease before any signs or symptoms appear. Asthmatic patient should regularly measure peak airflow with peak flow meter at home.

- Quit smoking as it is common with any other respiratory disease, smoking adversely affects asthmatics in several ways including an increased severity of symptoms, a more rapid decline of lung function and a decreased response to medications. Asthmatics who smoke require additional medications to control their disease. Smoking cessation and avoidance of second hand smoke is strongly indicated in asthmatics

- Drink8-10 glasses of water daily to keep your digestive system healthy and prevent constipation.

- Bronchitis- It is inflammation of main air passage of the lungs. Bronchitis may be short-lived (acute) or chronic, meaning that it lasts a long time and often reoccurs.

- Acute bronchitis may be caused by bacterial or viral infection. Bronchitis occurs more frequently in winter and more commonly in cold damp climates, commencing as common cold or inflammation of the nose, throat and sinuses, the inflammation may spread in to the chest.

- Chronic bronchitis is a long term condition. It is a degenerative disease. After repeated attacks of bronchitis, the walls of the bronchial tubes become thickened, inelastic and narrowed. The mucous membrane of the bronchi are permanently inflamed and the air ways become filled with tenacious sticky mucous.

- Symptoms of either type of bronchitis include cough that produces mucous, shortness of breath, wheezing, fatigue, fever and chest discomfort. Cigarette smoke including long term exposure to second hand smoke is the main cause of chronic bronchitis.

1.10.02.Pneumonia:- It is the illness of lungs in which the alveoli (microscopic air filled sacs of the lungs responsible for absorbing oxygen) become inflamed and are flooded with fluid. Pneumonia can result from variety of causes including infection with bacteria, virus, fungi and parasites. Pneumonia may also occur from chemical or physical injuries to the lungs or indirectly due to other medical illness such as lung cancer or alcohol abuse. Typical symptoms associated with pneumonia are cough, chest pain, fever and difficulty in breathing.

1.10.03. Pleurisy:- In this the normally smooth lining of lungs (the pleura) becomes rough. Typically, it causes sharp pain, almost always during the act of breathing. A rough grating sound called friction rub can be heard with the stethoscope. Pleurisy may develop due to a variety of causes. These include acute viral infection, pneumonia, rheumatoid arthritis, tuberculosis and pancreatitis.

1.10.04. Cough:- It is a sudden noisy explosion of air from the lungs. It is usually a reflex response of the body caused by an irritation in the throat or wind pipe. There are many possible causes of cough ranging from allergies to lung infection and cancer.

1.11. Digestive System:- The digestive system is body's power source. It breaks down food so that sugar, fats, proteins, vitamins, minerals and water can be absorbed into the blood, and used to provide energy for repair and growth. Anything the body cannot use is expelled as feces. Maintains a healthy weight, following a balanced diet and exercising regularly helps to keep the digestive system functioning.

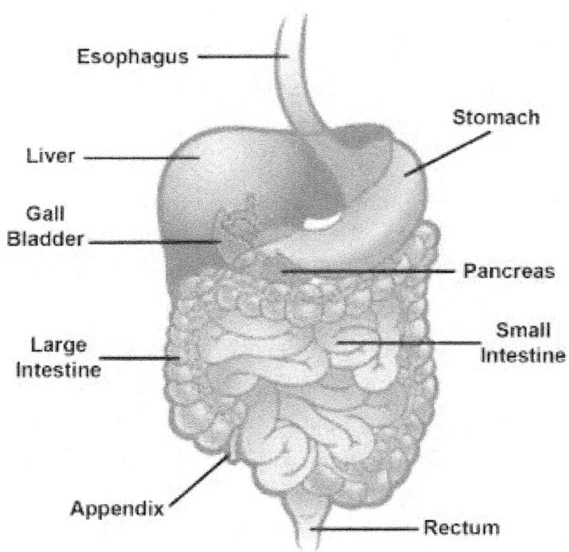

The digestive system consists partly of the digestive tract and partly of the digestive glands. The digestive tract is basically a long tube running from the mouth to the anus. The digestive glands, the liver and pancreas, make various chemicals needed to attack and break down the pieces of food we swallow.

1.11.01. The Digestive process: -

-The process of digestion starts in the mouth. Here the teeth work with the muscular tongue and saliva to cut, crush and mix food to be swallowed.

-After being chewed and swallowed, the food enters the esophagus. The esophagus is a long tube that runs from mouth to stomach. At the end of the oesophagus, a ring of muscle (sphincter) opens to allow food into the stomach. The food changes very little as it passes through the oesophagus.

-The stomach is a large sac like organ that churns food and bathes it in a very strong acid. It stores the food after the meal and then allows it bit by bit into next part of the digestive tract, the small intestine.

-After being in stomach, food enters the duodenum, the first part of the small intestine. It then enters the jejunum and ileum (the final part of the small intestine). In small intestine, bile produced by liver and stored in gallbladder and pancreatic enzymes helps in breaking down of food. Main function of small intestine is that of absorption. About 80% of the food is absorbed through the walls of small intestine.

-Following the small intestine, the next region of tract is large intestine. The large intestine has three parts-the caecum, colon and rectum. Here water is absorbed from the undigested remains and the result is semisolid feces. The feces are stored in the end of the large intestine, chiefly in the part called rectum. Finally the wastes are expelled at convenient intervals, through the last part of the tract, called the anus.

Many bowel problems revolve around the production of excess acid (ulcers, indigestion and heart burn), the upward escape of acid (hiatus hernia) and disordered movements of intestine (constipation, diarrhea and irritable bowel syndrome). The rapid turnover of the cells within the digestive tract predisposes to cancer, especially of the stomach and large intestine.

1.11.02. Liver:- The liver is the largest and most important metabolic organ in the body. It can be viewed as the body's major biochemical factory. It weighs about 1.4 kilo is reddish brown in color and is divided into four lobes of unequal size and shape. The liver lies on the right side of the abdominal cavity beneath the diaphragm. Liver performs as astonishingly large number of tasks that impact all the body systems.

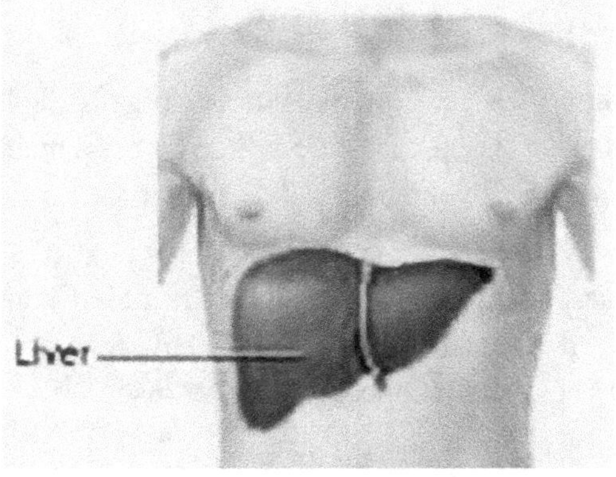

One of the major functions of the liver is secretion of bile. Liver secrets a remarkable 1 liter of bile every day, half of which is stored temporarily in the gall bladder. Bile is necessary for absorption of fat from food.

- The liver cells assimilate carbohydrates, fats and proteins. They convert glucose to its stored from glycogen, which is reconverted into glucose as the body requires it for energy. The ability of the liver to maintain proper level of glucose in the blood is called its glucose buffer function.

- The end products of the fat digestion, the fatty acids are used to synthesize cholesterol and other substances needed by the body. Excess carbohydrates and proteins are also converted into fat by the liver.

- Detoxification or degradation of body wastes and hormones as well as drugs, alcohol and other foreign compounds is done by liver.

- Urea, a waste product of protein breakdown, is produced by the liver, a process which removes poisonous ammonia from body fluids.

- Also the liver contains cells that catch and destroy bacteria and viruses from the intestine and so prevent them from gaining access to the rest of the body.

- Liver stores important minerals and vitamins including Vitamin A, D, K and B12.

- Some essential components of the blood are manufactured by the liver including about 95% of plasma proteins and blood clotting substances (fibrinogen and prothrombin).

The liver is among the few internal human organs capable of natural regeneration of lost tissue, as little as 25% of remaining liver can regenerate into a whole liver again.

1.11.03. Diseases of Liver: - With its huge blood supply and never ending activity, it is to be expected that liver is prone to disease. Hepatitis and cirrhosis are most common liver disorders.

1.11.04:1. Hepatitis: - It is an inflammatory disease of the liver that results from a variety of causes, including viral infection or exposure to toxic agents like alcohol. Hepatitis ranges in severity from mild, reversible symptoms to acute massive liver damage with possible imminent death resulting from acute liver failure.

Viral hepatitis now range from A to E. Hepatitis A is spread by mouth, usually by eating contaminated food. The virus causes fever, jaundice and abdominal discomfort which subside over a period of three to six weeks. Long term effects are rare and no treatment is needed. Other such as B and C are transmitted by sexual contact or through blood products and intravenous drug abuse. Mothers positive for hepatitis B almost always pass on the virus to the unborn baby. Internationally, hepatitis B is a major cause of chronic hepatitis, cirrhosis and liver cancer.

1.11.04:2. Cirrhosis:- It's a chronic liver disease in which normal liver cells are damaged and replaced by scar tissue, decreasing the amount of normal liver tissue. The most common cause of cirrhosis is alcohol abuse. Though it affects many organs, alcohol is especially harmful to the liver. Alcohol must be metabolized and the liver performs most of the job, suffering serious damage in the process. Not only does alcohol destroy liver cells, it also robs them of their ability to regenerate. Such co-factors as Hepatitis C virus can increase the risk of cirrhosis. If detected in early stages, cirrhosis can be treated. If not the liver hardens, shrivels and is unable to function, leading to death.

1.11.04.3. Tumors: - The majority of tumors within the liver spread there via the rich blood supply from cancer elsewhere, especially bowel tumors. This so called secondary liver cancer is often the way in which the people with cancer finally die. Worldwide primary cancer of liver is also common and often follows previous infection with Hepatitis B virus.

1.11.04.4. Jaundice: Jaundice is not a disease but a sign of some disease. Many diseases can cause jaundice including gallstones, various forms of hepatitis, tumor of the liver or pancreas and rarely cirrhosis of liver. In jaundice, the skin and whites of eyes turn yellow due to build up yellowish brown substance, bilirubin, in the blood, Bilirubin is a waste product formed when old red blood cells are broken down. Normally, it is extracted from the bloodstream by the liver, collects in gallbalder as bile, passes down the bile duct into the intestines and is excreted in the feces (Bilirubin colors and feces brown). The feces are no longer brown but chalky grey. In addition, bilirubin may darken the urine. Jaundice also causes severe itching of the skin. Jaundice can also appear if the exit for bile is obstructed, for example by a gallstone. Bilirubin accumulates in the bile and then overflows back into the blood stream. If you develop jaundice for any reason, you should visit a doctor immediately for a full examination.

1.11.05. Gall Bladder: - Just beneath the liver lies the gallbladder, a pear shaped sac about 3 inches long. The liver manufactures the bile while the

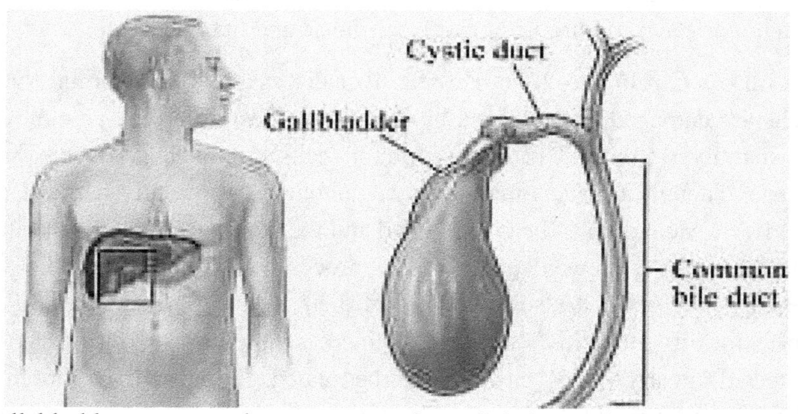

gall bladder stores and concentrates it until it is needed. Bile contains water, cholesterol, bile salts, protein and bilirubin. Bile works to emulsify fats, allowing them to be absorbed into the body, and is essential for absorption of important fat soluble vitamins. Among these are Vitamin A, which is necessary for good night vision and healthy skin and hair; vitamin D, which promotes healthy bones and teeth; vitamin E, which prevents the oxidation of unsaturated fats and vitamin K, a key component in normal blood clotting. Furthermore, bile acts as a deodorizer and a mild laxative.

1.11.05.1. Gall Stones: Sometimes the concentration of bile can cause problems for the gall bladder. If the bile becomes too concentrated, small particles may precipitate out to form gall stones. Gall stones can be as small as a grain of sand or as large as a golf ball. Gall stones are extremely common. 10%-20% of adult population has them and only a fraction of them causes symptoms. Women are twice as likely as men to suffer from gall stones, but in later life, there is a roughly equal chance of gall stones.

Most gall stones are silent. They lie within the gall bladder and are simply a chance finding on routine investigations. A stone obstructing the gall bladder causes severe upper right sided abdominal pain, which comes and goes in waves as strong muscular contractions try to overcome the obstruction. Pain is usually more after eating-especially after fatty food because fats in food provoke reflex contraction of gall bladder. If there is complete obstruction, infection of gall bladder invariably results after 24 hours causing fever and jaundice.

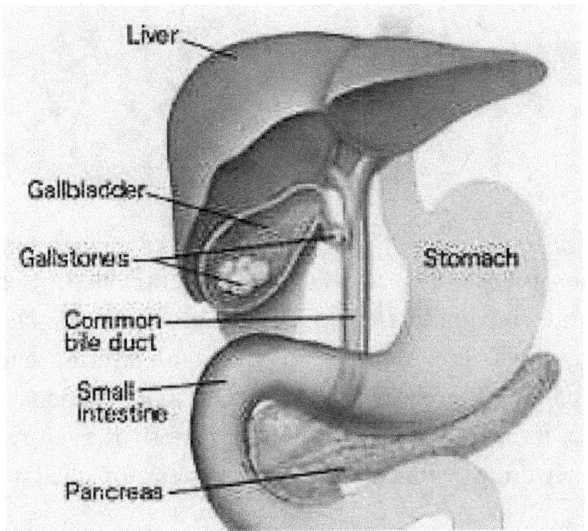

Obesity is a major risk factor for gall stones, especially in women.

A large clinical study showed that being even moderately overweight increases the risk for developing gall stones. Obesity tends to reduce the amount of bile salt in bile, resulting in more cholesterol. Obesity also decreases gall bladder emptying.

1.11.06. Peptic Ulcer:- Peptic ulcers include both gastric (stomach) and duodenal ulcers. Duodenal ulcers are three times more common than gastric ulcers and are common in 20-45 age groups. On the other hand, people with the gastric ulcers are likely to be over 50.

-The stomach secrets highly concentrated hydrochloric acid which begins the process of digestion and sterilizes the food. Thick mucus coats the walls of the stomach, protecting it from this acid. Despite the mucus coating of the stomach and duodenum, their linings can come under attack from this powerful acid. An ulcer is an area of the tissue that has been damaged by this acid.

-The vast majority of peptic ulcers are caused by infection with Helicobacter pylori bacteria. People living in unhygienic living

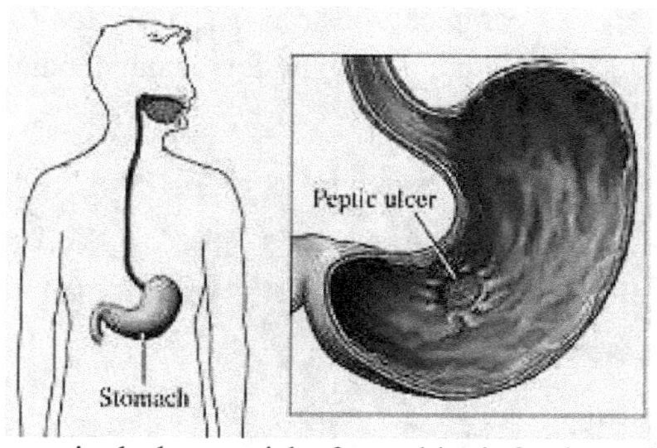

conditions are particularly at risk from his infection. Certain drugs irritate the protective lining of the stomach. NSAIDS (non-steroidal anti-inflammatory drugs) are used for treatment of arthritis and muscular aches and pains. These include aspirin, indomethacin, ibuprofen, diclofenac etc. If taken regularly for a long period, these drugs can cause ulcers by interfering with the defense system of the stomach and duodenum.

-There is also another factor which is perhaps as important in the causation of ulcer and that is dietary factor. In India, duodenal ulcer is seen most commonly in Kerala, Tamil Nadu and Punjab where the diet consists of greater quantities of chilies and spices. Apart from the direct injurious action on the mucosa, these substances act as stimulants for production of acid in the stomach in excessive quantities. Excessive consumption of alcohol and possibly caffeine predisposes to ulcers.

Although smoking itself is no longer thought to be an independent cause of peptic ulcers, it is known that tobacco smoking significantly impairs ulcer healing, so anyone who has an ulcer and smokes is advised to stop.

Stress is a contributing factor because it increases acid production. There may be a genetic factor since there often seems to be a family history of the condition.

Symptoms: Early symptoms of duodenal ulcer may be difficult to differentiate from what is vaguely termed as indigestion. One of the characteristic features of the condition is burning, gnawing pain in the pit of the stomach. There may be heartburn. The pain is aggravated by an empty stomach and is often relieved by eating. In later stages vomiting may occur. The two life threating complications of duodenal ulcer are bleeding from ulcer which leads to vomiting of blood and passing reddish black colored stools and a perforation which means bursting of the ulcer, thus releasing the stomach and duodenal contents into the peritoneal cavity leading to peritonitis.

To prevent ulcers from recurring, your doctor may advise you to make long term lifestyle changes such as reducing high levels of stress at work, giving up smoking and alcohol as appropriate.

1.11.07. Constipation: - Some people think they are constipated if they do not have a bowel movement every day. There is definition of constipation in the sense of how much, how often. Normal stool elimination may be three times a day or three times a week depending upon the person. If the bowels are opened only infrequently but without straining, there is no cause for concern whereas a daily struggle may indicate a problem.

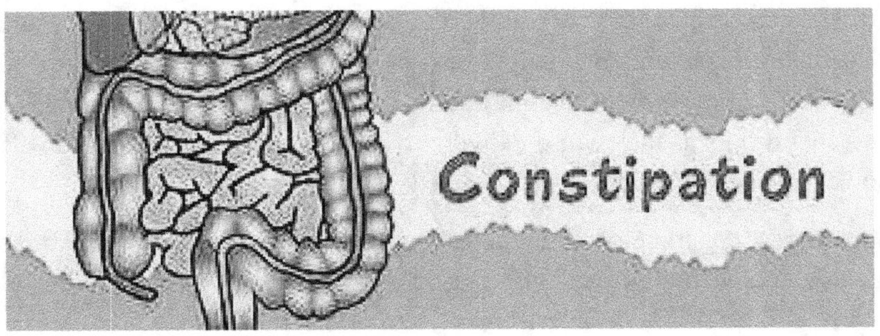

As the food moves through colon, the colon absorbs water from the food while it forms waste products or stool. Muscle contraction in the colon then pushes the stool towards the rectum. By the time stool reaches the rectum. It is solid because most water has been reabsorbed. Constipation occurs when the colon absorbs too much water or if the colon's muscle contractions are slow or sluggish, causing the stool to move through the colon too slowly. As a result, stools can become hard and dry. Most common cause of constipation is a diet low in fiber or a diet low in fiber or a diet high in fats such as cheese, eggs and meat. People who ignore the urge to have a bowel movement may eventually stop feeling the need to have one, which can lead to constipation. Some people delay bowel movement because they do not want to use toilet outside the home. Others ignore the urge because of emotional stress or because they are too busy. Children may postpone having a bowel movement because of stressful toilet training or because they do not want to interrupt their play. During pregnancy, women may be constipated because of the hormonal changes or because the uterus compresses the intestines. Aging may also affect bowel regularity because a slower metabolism results in less intestinal activity and muscle tone.

In most cases, dietary and life style changes will help relieve symptoms and help prevent them from recurring. A diet with enough fiber (20-35 Gms per day) helps the body from soft bulky stools. High fiber foods include beans, whole grains, fresh fruits and vegetables, sprouts, cabbage and carrot. For people prone to constipation, limiting foods that have little or no fiber such as ice cream, cheese, meats and processed foods is also important.

Other changes that may help treat and prevent constipation include drinking enough water and liquids such as fruit and vegetable juices and clear soups, engaging in daily exercise and reserving enough time to have a bowel movement. Avoid liquids that contain caffeine such coffee and cola drinks as they cause dehydration. In addition, the urge to have a bowel movement should not be ignored.

Sometimes, constipation can lead to complications. These complications include hemorrhoids (piles), caused by straining to have bowel movement or anal fissures (tears in the skin around the anus) caused when hard stool stretches the sphincter muscle. As a result, rectal bleeding may occur appearing as bright red steaks on the surface of the stool. Sometimes straining causes a small amount of intestinal lining to push out through the anal opening. This condition is called rectal prolapse.

1.12. Pancreas: -

Pancreas is a 15 to 20 cm long and flat gland. It produces a very effective enzyme which helps the food to breakdown in the intestine and has the ability to digest all the constituents of food.

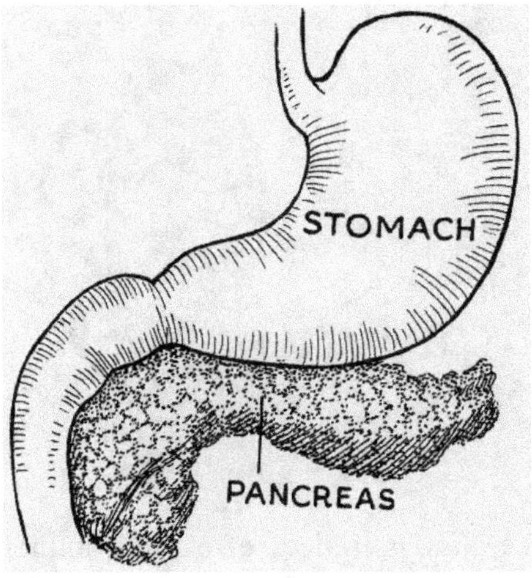

There are four types of enzymes in pancreatic juice that pass through a tube to duodenum. It contains enzymes and salts, which help in the digestion of protein, starch, sugar and fat. As soon as the food enters the mouth the taste buds convey signal to the brain through which the brain stimulate pancreas to produce digestive juices. This digestive juice contains sodium bicarbonate which neutralizes acid. The enzyme called amylopsin helps in digestion of carbohydrate whereas strep sin helps in the digestion of fat. The main enzyme which helps in the digestion of protein is called trypsin.

Apart from digestion this organ also produces hormones called insulin and glucagon. Insulin is such a hormone which reduces the level of sugar as and when it rises in the body. This hormone converts glucose into glycogen in the liver. These two hormones while working with each other control the supply of energy to the body.

1.13. Spleen: - It is an important organ of the body. It is located a little below and behind the stomach. Spleen is made of spongy tissue. Because of its spongy structure spleen can store a lot of blood. The spleen removes the pieces of those red blood corpuscles which get destroyed from the blood circulation. Spleen is also called the store house of excess quantity of blood. Red Blood corpuscles are found in compressed state. During emergency and sudden increase in work load the spleen contracts and pushes additional quantity of blood into normal blood circulation.

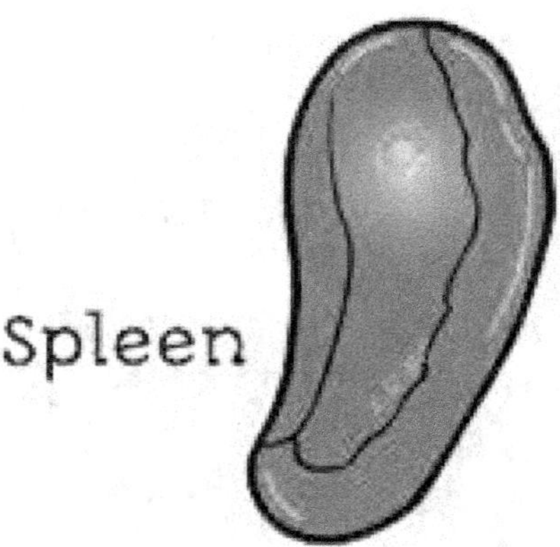

Thus whenever the body is in need of oxygen, millions of Red Blood Corpuscles, which are completely filled with oxygen, Reach for its help.

1.14. Excretory System:

The process of wear and tear keeps taking place in some cells of tissues. They get continuously repaired in accordance with the set mechanism in the body.

The food provides vigor and heat that makes these actions possible. Many ailments keep cropping up in the body due to slow metabolism of food and destruction of cells. Persistence of these ailments in the body for a long time could be detrimental: therefore, there are certain organs which keep evicting these virulent undesirable substances that in the body. Some of the undesirable substances that are there in the body are solid state; some are in liquid whereas some are in gaseous state. Kidney, skin and lung are the organs throwing out these undesirable substances from the body. Of these, Kidney is most important organ from the point of view of expulsion of waste substances.

Major organs: Kidney, Ureter, bladder, urethra.

Main function: Carries out the function of blood purification. The blood, while circulating, when it reaches the kidney, non-essential elements

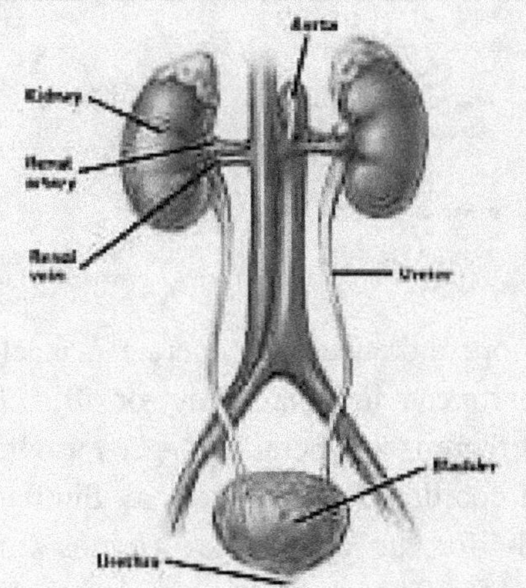

such as salt, extra water which are called urine are passed to urinary bladder by the kidney. The urine is then thrown out of the body from urinary bladder through urinary system.

There are two kidneys in our body out of which two 10 to 12 inches long tubes originate one end of which remains connected with kidney, while with the other end is connected to urinary bladder. These tubes are called ureters. In each kidney there are roughly 10 lac tiny sieves. Roughly 20 lac sieves are continuously engaged in the process of purification of blood. Through this nearly 1.5 liters of water, 30 grams of urea and 300 grams of other substances are ejected out of the body in a single day.

1.15. Nervous System:

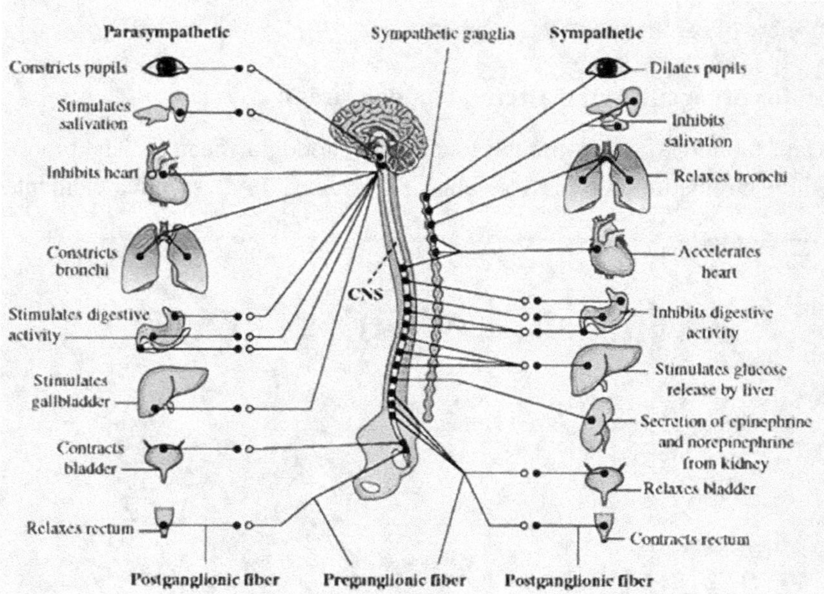

An operator needs to operate a machine properly. There are separate departments in a big factory or office for performing different functions. But there is a general manager for overall monitoring of all departments and coordination among them. Similarly, there is an operator in human body for the conduct of various functions. Nervous System is that operator. This special system has a place in the body which is meant to bring about coordination among the functions of various mechanisms in the complex mechanism called body. There are special organs for carrying out various functions viz. „moving, seeing, taking food, etc. Connected with all these organs is network of fine threads which pervades the whole body. These threads are called nerves and the network formed by them is called nervous system. These nerves combine together to form nervous system which remains connected with the brain. The nervous system co -ordinates each and every function and rules the whole body. In its absence all the organs in the body are rendered inactive. Controlling all the voluntary and involuntary actions and receiving all the stimuli and conveying them to the brain is function of this system. The function of nervous system is not confined to memory, discretion and knowledge alone, but it is an instructional force which makes quick adjustment possible in response to change in the internal and external conditions of all organs of the body. Man is responsive to the influences exerted by the external environment. Body gets affected by the physical and chemical changes constantly taking place in the external environment. The body definitely reacts to these changes in some way or the other. As soon as a thorn pricks our leg, the protoplasm in the cells of our leg feel the sensation, the signal of which reaches the brain through special nerves. There is a sensation in the cerebral cells as soon as the signal is received by them. The stimulus generated because of this reverts back to the cells in the leg. At that point there occurs a change in the cells and the leg automatically moves away from that place. Thus the impact of external environment is no confined to any local cells in the body; rather the whole physical actions are affected by it.

1.15.01.Nerves:- The functions which are performed in the nervous system and various components of it are, in fact, the functions performed by the nerve cells lying there. Just as an organ like liver is made up of numerous tiny units of liver cells, likewise, nervous system too is formed by units called nerve cells based on functions and features; there are two main components of nervous system.

1.15.01:01. Voluntary Nerves:- All the nerve fibers in this zone are found in voluntary muscles. Sensations are carried to brain by the fibers. We receive different sensations through this technique and inspire ourselves to work as per the outer atmosphere. We move our hands or legs as per our will.

1.15.01:02. Involuntary Nervous System:- Nerve fibers of this section go to the lungs, urinary, bladder, uterus, stomach, heart and to different glands. We cannot control its action. Sensations are carried by these nerves to brain through internal organs. These nerves perform on their own that is why they are called automatic nerves.

1.15.01:03. Afferent/Sensory Nerves:- Nerves which accept sensations through other parts or outer layer and carry them to central nervous system are afferent nerves.

1.15.01:04. Efferent/Motor Nerve:- Nerve which carry impulses from central nerves system to muscles or any organ, tissue are called efferent nerve.

There are two parts of nervous system-

1.15.01:05. Central Nervous System: Formed by the brain and the spinal cord.

Peripheral Nervous System: Formed by 12 pairs of cranial nerves and 31 pairs of spinal nerves.

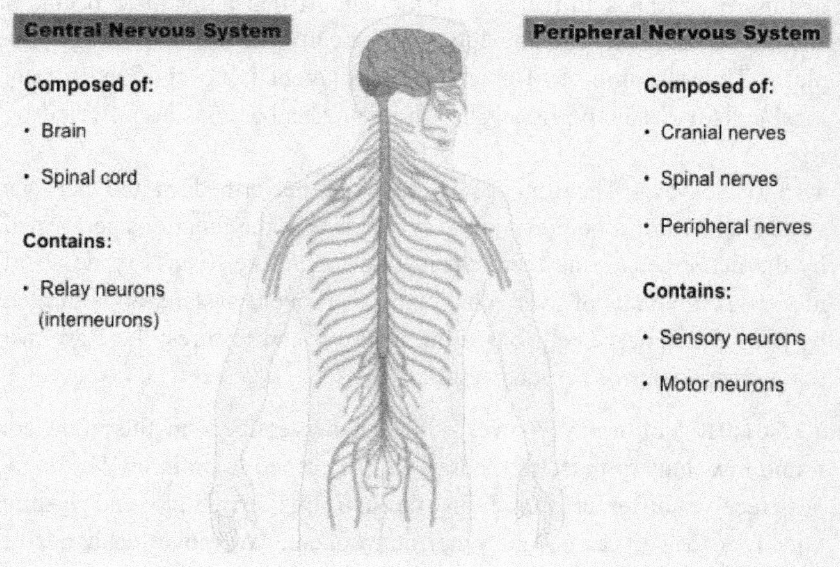

1.16.   Reproductive System:- Copulation is necessary among different sexes of living beings for reproduction. There are separate reproductive organs in male and female bodies for reproduction. They are known as reproductive organs. These organs are different among men and women.

1.16.01.Men: Main Organs:-

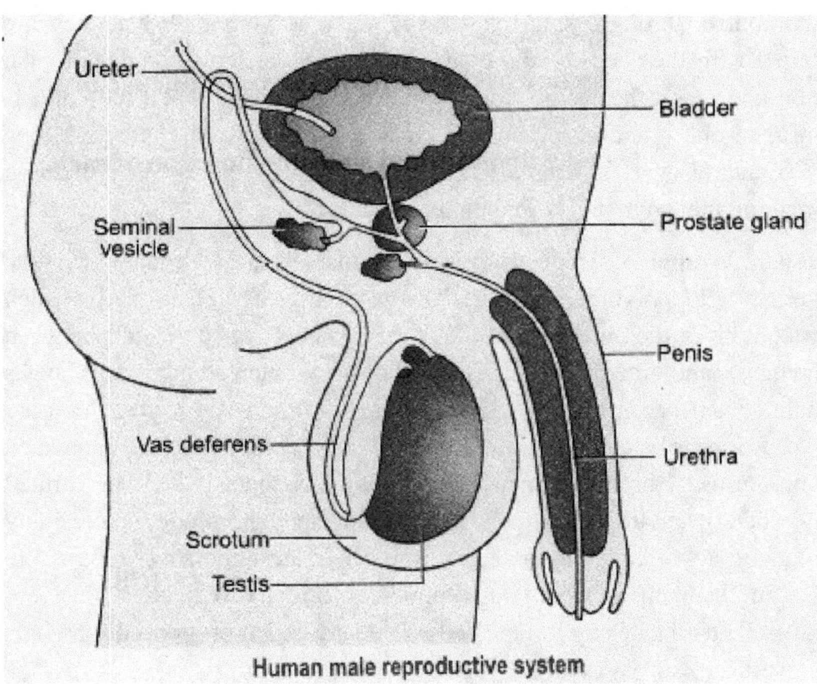

Human male reproductive system

Testes, vas deferens, seminal vesicle, prostate and penis. Testes are situated outside the male body in a Sac. They are two in number and oval in shape. There are nine or ten compartments in each testis which are full of sperms. There are about 1,000 veins in one testis. Because they in the form of a bunch, they are accommodated in a small place. They meet at the back of the glands. After that they combine together to form two or three closely knit chains which end in forming sperm carrying tube. This is a six meter long tube which is attached to the back of testes. One end of the tube is in the testes while the other end forms the sperm carrying tube. Both these tubes pass through the cavity in the abdomen and meet near urinary track in two small Sacs, which store sperms. From these two tiny and thin tubes begin and pass under urinary track and open near kidneys. They are called exit tubes. Through them the sperms are discharged. Under glands and on both sides of the urinary tract there are two small glands like beans which are called Coupler gland.

The sperms are produced in the testes. From there they are carried during intercourse, through penis in the vagina of a woman. When they are joined with the seeds of the ovary, which are carried through fallopian tube and reach the womb, the woman gets pregnant. Then the child is born. In one intercourse about 20-30 lac sperms are discharged. Along with them sugar, calcium. Citrate etc. are also there which help in breaking the ovum and complete the process.

1.16.02.Women's Reproductive Organs:- Main Organs: Vagina, uterus, fallopian tube, ovaries. The vagina is a tube of cells which extends from the outer part to the uterus. This acts as a conduit between the uterus and outer part. This is a part of the women's body that receives male sexual organ and also gives birth. Like the male testes, there are two ovaries, of shape of almond and brown in color. They are connected with uterus by broad ligament. There are many septas which are formed by fiber. Its main function is to develop many hormones excessively affecting a woman's physical function. There are innumerable immature ova in the ovaries which are known as primary ova cells. Ova are covered on all sides by follicle cells. They are called primordial follicles.

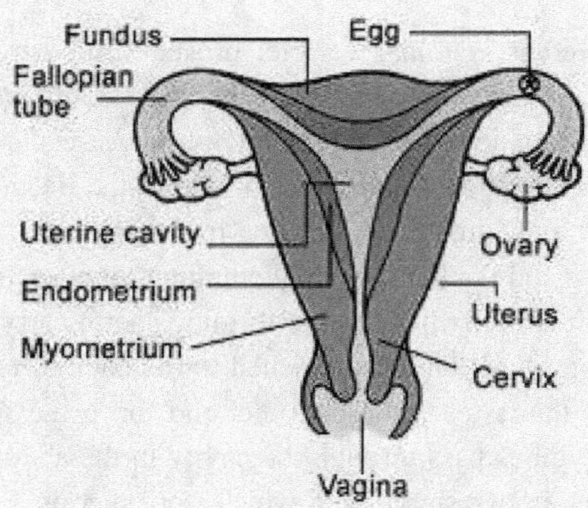

In childhood the ovary in every girl contains thousands of ova. On an overage only four to five hundred of them mature. Normally the form in the outer layer is germinal epithelium. Among the cells only the centra cell makes ova. After forming the liquid inside the cell at the Centre gets separated from the outer layer along with the cells in its contact. The distance between them increases which is filled by liquor foliiculi. The volume of liquid increases along with the size of the sheath and it begins moving towards the bottom of the gland. Liquor filicide slowly gets ripened and rise is noticed on the outer layer. Primordial follicles cells are ripened in 10-14 days. When they reach the outer layer of ovary, there is tension in primordial Follicles which results in its breaking. Because of this the cells come out of ovaries and enter the peritoneal cavity. Due to exit of the cell, there is little bleeding. This is called ovulation. This process takes place after 13 to 17 days after menstruation. The place, occupied by the chrysalis is filled by clotted blood. Slowly particles of a yellow oily substance are collected there. The place, which is empty after the chrysalis are discharged the grarion follicle is filled by new crowd of cells, which is yellow in color. It is known as corpus luteum. The cells go from peritoneal cavity through fallopian tube processes. The cell in the tube also help in their progress. If the sperms join the ovum in the tube they are fertilized and enter the uterus. There it takes a form of a fetus and pregnancy starts. If the ovum does not join the sperm then it dies and is thrown out of the body via menstrual discharge.

1.17. Ear: - The organ through which we hear is known as Ear.

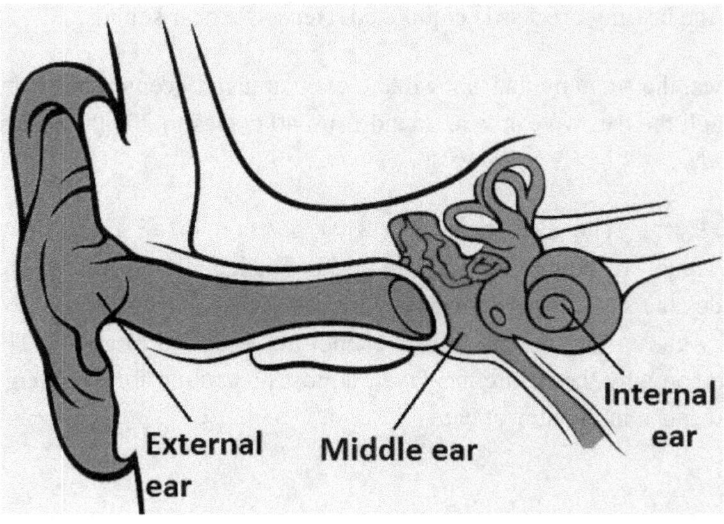

1.17.01.Outer Ear: - The visible part is called the pinna. It is composed of a thin plate of yellow elastic cartilage, covered with integument and connected to the surrounding parts of ligaments and muscles. There is a ditch which goes to the head. It is called hearing tube.

1.17.02.Middle Ear: - It is a small bowl and has a screen on outside wall, known as ear drum. There are small bones Malleus, Anvil and Stapes which are, joined in a chain.

1.17.03.Inner Ear: - The portion of the ear located within the temporal bone that is involved in both hearing and balance plus includes the semicircular canal vestibule and cochlea etc. It is also called internal ear. It has a membranous labyrinth. It has three half-moon shaped tubes, cochlea etc. Cochlea resembles a shell. There are many tiny holes in it from where veins go inside. Cochlea has an auditory canal. The other end of the vein is connected with the brain. The waves made by any noise in the air, are collected by the outer part of pinna. They go through hearing auditory canal and hit ear drum which creates vibrations in it. The ear drum is connected with the central ear. Therefore the air in central ear gets vibrated. After that the waves of noise reach membranous labyrinth, first to cochlea and then to auditory canal. This causes nervous impulse. This nervous impulse is then sent to the hearing Centre in other head. Thus the hearing process is completed. Hence we hear sounds.

Besides, the semicircular tubes in the ear help us in keeping our balance. Through the ear, we can hear sound from 40 cycles to 20,000 cycles per second.

1.18. Eye:- The eye occupies a vital position in all five organs of knowledge. It helps us in gaining knowledge about everything. It includes the sensitivity connected with high rays, shape, distance, color, density etc. In fact its importance cannot be described in words. This is the reason why the nature has taken utmost precaution for its safety and maintenance in the utmost care.

Both the camera and the eye have a lens to focus the image on a light sensitive surface in the camera is the role or plate of film. In the eye it is a layer of light sensitive nerve cells called the retina. In the camera the distance between the lens and the film usually can be changed to keep the image in focus for objects both near and far away. In the eye, the shape of the lens is changed automatically by small muscles, so that we can see clearly objects at various distances.

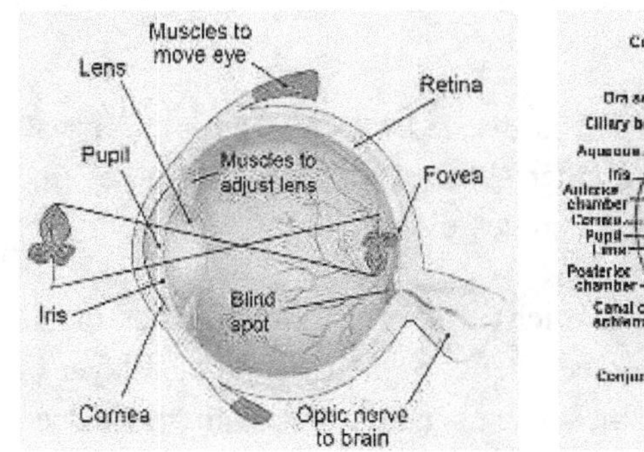

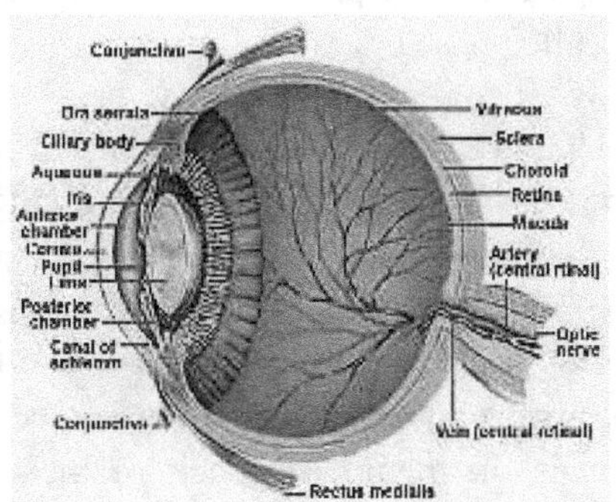

A further similarity between the eye and the camera is that of iris, the curtain at the front of the eye that can be opened or closed to permit various amount of light to pass through the lens. In the camera, the iris may be controlled by energy from photoelectric cell or it may be adjusted by hand. Iris by the action of tiny muscles it contains. The iris of eye adjusts automatically to change light intensity, again by the action of tiny muscles it contains. The opening in the iris of the eyeball is protected by a smooth, transparent layer of tissue called conjunctiva. A similar membrane covers the inner surfaces of the eyelids. The eyelids also contain dozens of tiny tarsal glands that secrete an oil to lubricate the surface of the eyeball and eyelids. Still further protection is provided by the lacrimal gland, located at the outer edge of the eye socket. It secretes tears to clean the protective membrane and keep it moist.

The innermost layer of eyeball, the retina, itself made up of eight layers of nerve tissue. Most of the layers contain nerve fibers. But the layer most directly involved in vision contains specialized nerve cells called rods and cones. The rods are more sensitive to light than the cones. The cones other hands are sensitive to colors. When we are trying to see an object at night, perhaps by moonlight we depend upon the rods. The faint amounts of light passing through the lens fall upon the retina and stimulate the rods which transmit through the optic nerve. The message that produce the visual image in the brain.

1.19. Nose:- The organ which helps us in smelling anything is called nose. The outer part of the nose is known as external nose and inner part is called nose cave.

1.19.01. External Nose:- This part is divided into two parts by a wall and they are called nostrils. The inner sides of these walls are covered with mucus. There is anet of tiny blood vessels.

1.19.02. Nose Caves: The part which is seen behind the nostrils is known as nose cave. There is a screen between them. There is a layer of mucus on them. The back of the nose is connected with the throat. Therefore sometimes while drinking water or while laughing water enters from nose to throat.

1.19.03: Function of Nose:

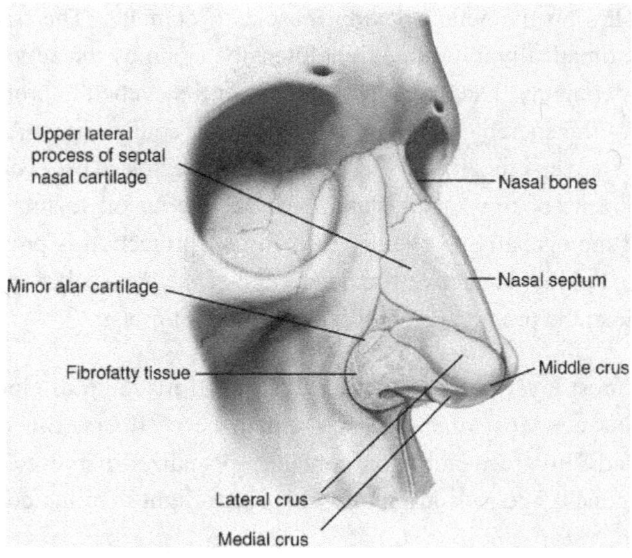

We smell through nose. There are hairs inside nostrils. When we breathe, the dust particles and germs are prevented from entering because of these hairs. When the air passing through nose enters the lungs, it becomes warm because of mucus covered hair. If the air is not warmed then veins will become swollen and it will give rise to cold. There are many glands in the nostrils that produce mucus. This keeps the nose wet. When a person suffers from cold the glands produce more of this.

1.20. Tongue: - The organ which helps us in determining taste is called tongue. The upper layer of the tongue is dry and there are taste buds over it. When anything touches the tongue, taste determining cell in the tongue are stimulated. They send a message through taste buds, to the taste Centre in the brain. The tongue plays a vital role of taste as well as it helps in creating sound.

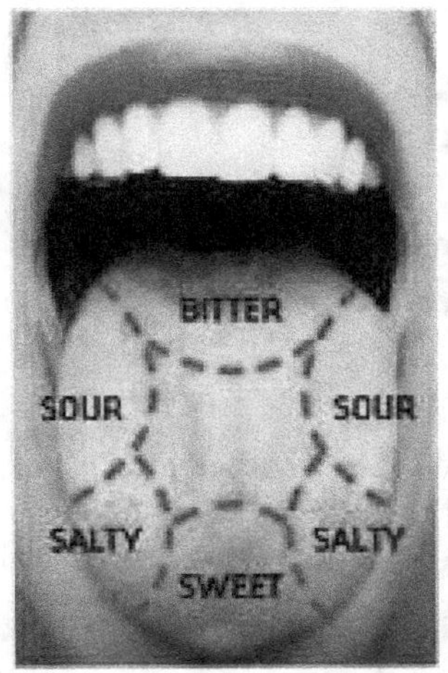

Functions:

-To assist in chewing.
-Swallowing- It helps in swallowing the chewed mouthful in entering esophagus.
 -Flowing- Keeps mouth wet by secreting saliva in it.
-Sense of touch.
-Taste Knowledge.
-Helps in creating sound.

1.21. Skin: - All other organs of the body are located at a particular place. They work in a definite field. But the skin has an expanded field. Besides touch, it helps in determining fever, pain pressure. Hot or cold, light or heavy, rough or smooth etc. are known through the skin. Small areas are spread throughout the skin for this all over the skin. There is a net of the ends of nerve fibers in the skin. They are the end organs for a particular sensation and are known as receptors. The points when touched sense the information of touch are called touch points. Similarly the points which if touched experience fever, cold or pain are called fever, cold points. There is difference among different points in numbers. The skin is an outer cover which protects internal organs and provides grace to the body. The thickness of the skin is between 1mm and 4 mm. it is thinnest on the lips and thickest on the soles of the feet and palms of hand.

1.21.01.Main functions:
- Protection
- General Sensitivity
- Controlling Fever
- Absorbing
- Extraction
- Production of liquids
- Water level control.
- Chemical Work
- Acid- Alkaline Balance
- Preservation acts
- Gas exchange
- Showing symptoms which helps to diagnosis

1.21.02.One Square Centimeter of skin contains;
- 100 Sweat Glands
- 10 hair
- 30 lac Cells
- 12 sensory Apparatuses for heat

- 2 Sensory Apparatuses of cold
- 200 nerve ending to record pain
- 25 Tactile Corpuscles
- 1 yard blood vessels
- 4 yard Nerves
- 3000 sensory cells at the end of the nerve fibers.

1.21.03.Sensory Organ Skin:

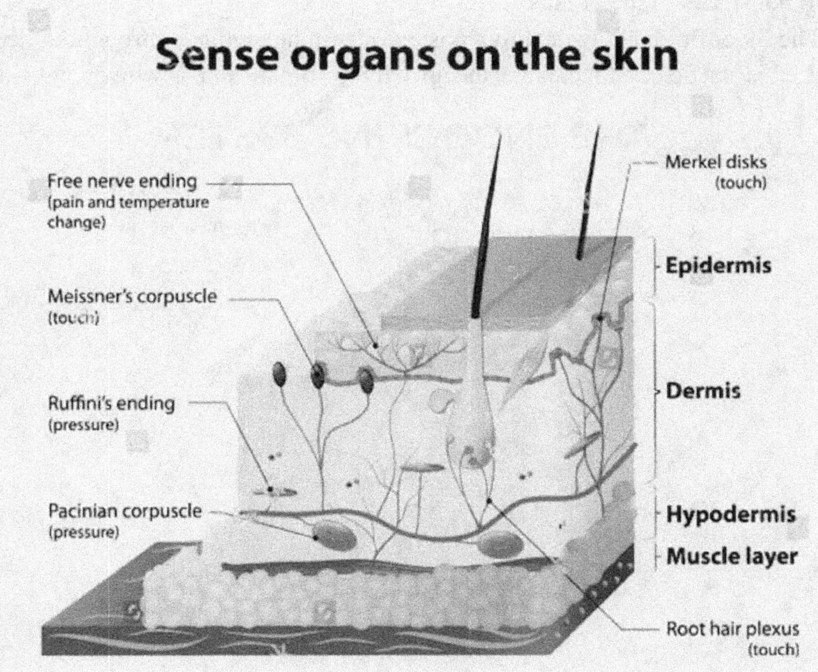

- Pain-Touch-Heat-Pressure-Traction-Cold-Tickle

ENDOCRINE GLANDS

There are many chemical activities which take place in the body continuously at the same time and many glands produce different chemical agents. The chemical substances produced by glands are made for a particular function. They are called hormones. These liquids are mixed in blood and give stimulation of some kind. They exchange message among various organs of the body. Small quantity is sufficient to boost acts of the organs.

The inner fluid, equivalent to a postage stamp in a woman throughout her life, is sufficient to change the girl into woman and a woman into a

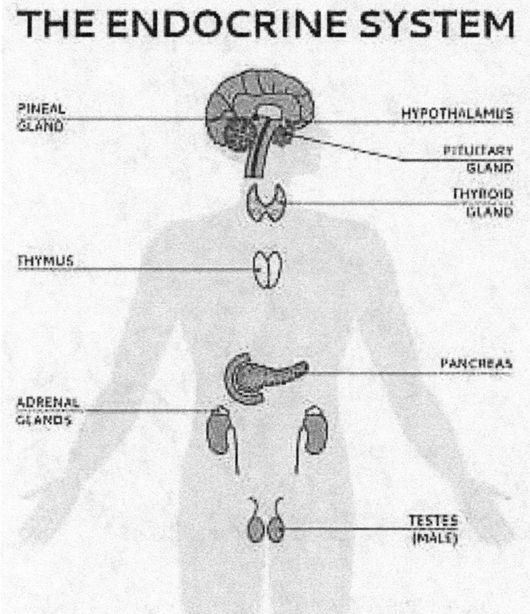

mother. The thyroid gland, throughout the life, produces only a teaspoonful inner fluid but its shortage causes dwarfness in a child or swelling of body in adult. There are two types of glands in the body.

2.01. Exocrine Glands:- The glands produce secretion that sent by ducts. They are called exocrine glands. E.g. sweat glands, salivary, lacrimal, gastric glands, etc.

2.02. Endocrine Glands:- The glands which produce hormones and send it directly to be mixed in the blood as follows

2.03. Pituitary:- This gland controls air and space in the body. This gland is like a king of all glands and sends order to all other glands. It controls will-power, sight, hearing, memory and sense of discrimination. It also rectifies the fault of other glands.

When it is predominant, it helps people to become great geniuses, eminent literary men, poet, scientists, philosophers and lovers of mankind.

As the gland controls the growth of the body, it's overworking leads to make people physically big in size, while its insufficient functioning may result in making them dwarfs.

This gland also governs the growth of the mind-brain. This gland may be damaged due to fear or injury or sometimes, due to tension during pregnancy. This also leads to the malfunctioning of other glands. And that results in giving birth to mentally retarded children. So if this problem of mentally retarded children is to be solved, the pregnant women during their pregnancy should take treatment on all endocrine glands and damage to fetus. Further it is observed that in those children where gland is not working sufficiently, they tend to become mean, heartless, mischievous, tend to become bullies, liar and disobedient. They are even ready to steal. With proper treatment of this gland, in most cases the parents and teachers will get amazing results. As this gland and pineal gland are situated in the head, it is harmful to hit the children on the head.

2.04. Pineal Gland:- It acts as an organizer and controller of all glands. It controls the development of glands and regulates them. Malfunctioning of this gland leads to high blood pressure, awakening of premature sex glands even sex delinquency, moreover it controls the potassium/sodium balance in the body and so the malfunctioning leads to excessive retention of fluids in the body which is mistaken for a serious kidney problem. It controls the proper flow of Cerebro Spinal Fluid and thus keeps all the glands and body vitalized, strong and healthy.

It is also known as primitive third eye. The predominance of this gland generates a sense of sublimity helping men grow into saints, endowed with divine qualities. These people have great wisdom and tenderness of heart, but also strong will power and so are not affected by physical sufferings or sorrow.

2.05. Lymph Gland:- Although they are not endocrine glands, because of their importance they have been included here. They control the immune defense system of our body, prevent the formation of pus on any cut or boil on the body and quickly heal the wounds. These glands help clear the toxins from the body, clear the dead cells from the system. But when such toxins and dead cells are in excess in the body these glands have to overwork and so they become weak and tender. At such time when you press on the reflex points of these glands and it pains. If such pain continues, it means that these glands are not able to stop the malignant growth forming from toxins and dead cells. As such the first symptom to detect cancer even at a very early stage is to find out about any pain on this gland.

2.06. Thymus Gland:- This is very important gland and can be considered as a God Mother of the child. It protects the growing young child against any disease. Once the body is fully developed, this gland shrinks and stops its activities. However if for some reason, if it becomes active, it produces dullness and general fatigue leading to total inactiveness.

2.07. Thyroid/Parathyroid Glands:- These glands play an important role in the development of child's body. As they digest calcium and eliminate poison, toxins they assist in controlling of the heat of the body and thus maintains the child's health. If these glands do not function properly, it leads to weakness, diseases even twisting muscles, leading to rickets and convulsions and so the development of a child is retarded. The child becomes fat and dull. Similarly, the overworking of this gland leads to overgrowth, bulging eyes, goiter, protruding Adam's apple and tendency to become bully. Even after puberty, if this gland does not function properly, it leads to problem of calcification (stone). This gland controls the elements of air and so the lungs and heart.

It also builds human qualities like affection, love, capacity for high thinking and concentration leading to self-control and balanced temperament, purity of heart and unselfishness. When it is degenerated a person becomes mentally unsteady, too talkative and ungrateful. When this gland damaged along with sex glands, the women during pregnancy and after child birth or removal of ovaries, tend to become plummy and put on weight around the abdominal and waist.

2.08. Ovary-Testes-Sex Gonad Glands:- These glands maintain the unbroken chain of procreation. They also regulate water element and also nerves, cells, flesh, bones, bone marrow and semen. They also regulate digestion of phosphorous in the body and thus regulate heat of the body.

2.09. Pancreas Gland:- These glands regulate digestion of sugar-glucose in the body by creating insulin. In modern times due to excessive use of sugar, (not the natural sugar in cereals-fruits-milk-honey-which is easily digestible) it has become more necessary to look after the proper functioning of this gland.

Further as per the latest research, it has been observed that over functioning of this gland leads to low B.P., Migraine and a times creates more desire for sweet food and sweet drinks leading sometimes even to alcohol

2.10. Adrenal Gland:- This gland controls and regulates the fire element of the body and so controls spleen, liver and gall bladder and assist creation of biles and digestive juices. Qualities like keenness of perception, untiring activity, and the drive to action, inner energy and courage are due to proper functioning of gland. It also intensifies the flow of blood helps proper oxygenation and develops organizing power, leads to leadership. It plays an important part in character building of a child.

In case of disorder of this gland, person abuse their natural vigor to satisfy their lust or antisocial activities. They suffer from sense of vain glory and are conceited, become extremely restless, impatient and short tempered. They cannot control diet and suffer stomach problems and blood pressure. Such persons become fearful, timid and lose vigor to face problems in life.

Endocrine Glands-Regulators of The Body

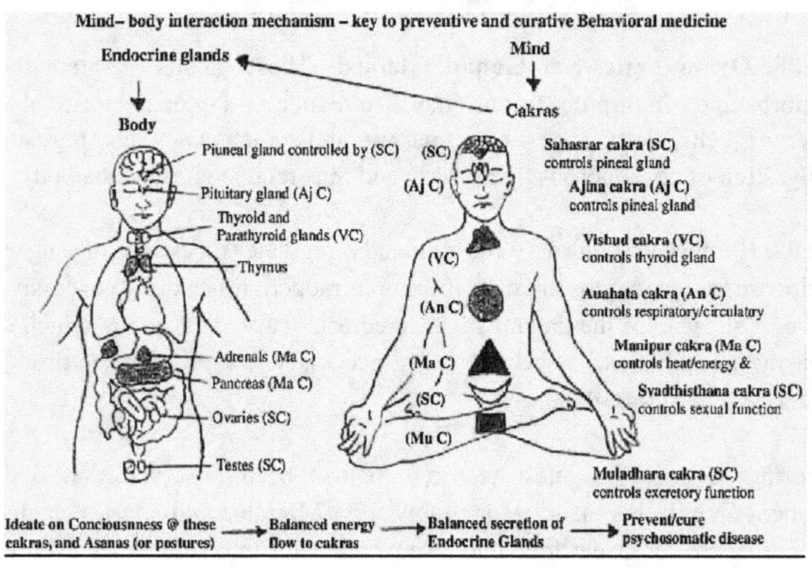

Name of Chakra	Equivalent Endocrine Gland	Its Function/Working
1. Sahastrar	Pineal (Point No. 4)	Regulates water balance; acts as a manager of all glands, controls Cerebro spinal fluid and sex desire. Stimulates the growth of nerves.

2.	Ajna	Pituitary (Point No. 3)	Controls air and space. It's like KING of all glands: controls growth of body and brain power and also memory.
3.	Vishudha	Thyroid/Parathy roid (Point No. 8)	Controls air- so lungs and heart; controls Temperature regulation,
4.	Anahat	Thymus (Point No. 38)	Acts as Godmother till child reaches puberty i.e. 12 to 15 years of age.
5.	Manipur	Adrenal & pancreas (Point No. 28 & 25)	Controls fire and production of digestive juices. Regulates blood and sugar levels. Controls stress-activeness and character building, controls sodium and water balance.
6.	Swadhisthan	Solar Plexus (Point No. 29)	Controls "Apan Vayu" and so regulates the movements of stool and urine, also controls all organs below the diaphragm.
7.	Mooladhar	Sex/Gonads (Point No. 11 to 15)	Controls water phosphorous content-Produces Sex hormones.

Functions & Effects of the Malfunctioning of Endocrine Glands

S. No.	Name of Gland	Functions	Effects of Malfunctioning
1	Thymus Gland	Protect the child up to the age of 15 years	Child gets sick. In case the gland becomes active later on, it brings dullness
2	Pineal Gland	Controls sex system and water of body and is a primitive eye.	Premature sex development, increase in water content, high B.P.
3	Pituitary Gland	It is the king of glands and controls the other glands. Governs the brain and development of the body.	Body becomes dwarfish or bulging. Produces mental retardation. Child becomes a bully, or a lair and disobedient.
4	Thyroid & Para-Thyroid Glands	Parathyroid gland controls digestion of calcium in the body, also controls the developments of the body.	Underworking leads to rickets, convulsion, and teeth problem, twisting of muscles, fatness and dullness. Overworking leads to over growth, bulging of the eyes., stone in kidney, etc.
5	Adrenal Gland	Controls production of biles and controls the liver and flow of blood pressure and also molds character.	Underworking leads to dullness, timidness, less energy, less oxygenation. Overworking leads to high BP, migraine, headache, Less bile leads to acidity and vomiting and severe headache.

6	Pancreas	Controls the digestion of sugar in the body, and digestive juices	Underworking leads to diabetes and overworking leads to low BP, dizziness and even to alcoholism through Hypoglycemia (Shortage of sugar)
7	Ovaries, Testes & Sex Glands	Digestion of phosphorus and heat of the body, attractiveness and productive side of the life.	Reproductive organs are damaged, problems of less or more menses, self- abuse, loss of heat leading to development of fat, un attractiveness of the body. Less/more sex desire.
8	Lymph Gland	Stops formation of pus and prevents germs	Disease called lymphocytosis leads to increase in blood sugar.

ACUPRESSURE

The menace of spurious drugs, the dangerous side effects of numerous medicines, the alarming figures of various diseases and above all costly medical treatment has remained a matter of serious concern for a majority of our people. I developed a strong inclination for a natural system which could extend the much needed cure to patients promptly, effectively.

There are many therapies known by names like Acupressure, Acupuncture, Zone Therapy, Reflexology, Shiatsu, Pointed Pressure Therapy, Contact Therapy, Concentrated Massage and Sujok Therapy is probably the oldest system of natural treatment in the world, based on the scientific technique of massage or pressure.

How, when and where this system originated lacks consensus but on the basis of certain ancient documents, it is assumed that Acupressure and Acupuncture, which works on the similar theory, were first conceived by Indian thinkers in primitive times. It was from here that the knowledge of these sciences disseminated to certain other countries through students, pilgrims and tourists. Research in Russia has endorsed this contention. On the basis of this research, it is said that the art and science of Acupuncture originated in India, not in China, as it is believed by most people in the world. This astounding revelation is made in the publication Indian Medicines in Ancient Russian treatment of diseases by N.A. Bogoyavlensky published in 1956 by the Gosudarstbennoye Izdatelstvo Meditsinkoi Literaturi (State Publishing House of Medical Literature), Leningrad Department.

According to Bogoyavlensky, one of the prominent scholars of China of VIIth century, Heun Tsang spent many years in Nalanda University in India. On his return to his country, he wrote a book in which he described in details the teaching work done in Nalanda University, particularly in the medical science. Another prominent scholar from China, I. Tzin who visited India in 673 A.D. also studied in Nalanda University for many years. In his works, Tzin described the customs of

Indian people, their clothes, food and occupations. He calls India a "Noble Province." He also mentioned that the Indians are imparting medical knowledge to the Chinese viz the complete art of treatment by pricking now called Acupuncture. He also confirmed the flourishing of various branches of medical science in India. Chinese translations of many Indian Manuscripts on philosophy, astronomy, mathematics and medical science have been preserved in various libraries in China till to date. From China, Indian writings on medicine also circulated to Tibet, and other countries.

Bogoyavlensky book also contains an interesting and revealing illustration which shows various points and areas in human body for purpose of curative cauterization and Acupuncture. This illustration dates back to the first century A.D. and was procured from Eastern India. These early writings undoubtedly establish India's pioneering role in the field of Acupressure and Acupuncture. Interestingly, reflexology historian Christine Issel has mentioned that certain traditional paintings of the feet of Hindu God Vishnu are covered in symbols coinciding with reflex points, which corroborate that acupressure, was widely practiced in earlier times in India.

Mr. Stanley Burroughs in his book "Healing for the Age of Enlightenment" has tried to authenticate that this sort of medical treatment was known and practiced in many parts of ancient India.

Popular of all complimentary therapies and nine to ten percent of the population of that country has tried this system to their satisfaction.

Japan has taken a lead in developing and popular sing a distinct type of pressure therapy called "Shiatsu", which is also based on the principles of acupressure. In Japanese language, the word SHI means finger and ATSU means pressure. Prof. Sir Park Jae Woo, a South Korean by birth, who has set up his academy in Moscow, gave Su-Jok system of treatment to the world in the year 1986 which has roots in acupressure.

In recent times, immense interest has been shown in reflexology by certain qualified professionals in Europe, U.S.A., Canada, Thailand,

Singapore, Malaysia, Germany, and Middle East including India, the place of its origin. Stephanie Rick in his book "The Reflexology Workout" has mentioned that in Europe nearly six thousand medical personnel combine reflexology as a part of their healing process these days. The number of such practitioners is increasing gradually. More and more people are now taking deep interest in this system. In view of its multifarious qualities, acupressure has now become one of the most popular systems of natural treatments in many countries.

Acupressure and Acupuncture Similarities & Dissimilarities:

Acupressure and Acupuncture are both ancient therapies. As mentioned earlier these systems were first conceived and practiced by Indian Physicians and from here these reached China and many other countries. In the present context, Chinese sages are credited for developing and widely practicing these natural models of treatment.

Acupressure is an amalgamation of two Latin words, Acu + Pressure. Acu means needle and pressure indicating pressure, thus, giving the impression that the treatment is through the pressure of needles. In the practice, its method of treatment is not through needles but by pressing certain reflex points in hands, feet and other parts of the body, with thumbs, fingers or some gadgets especially prepared for this purpose.

Acupuncture is also derived from two Latin words, Acu + Puncture. Acu means needle and puncture, thus conveying the meaning- treatment by pricking needles. Human body is endowed with a number of spots called acupuncture points. These points when stimulated by needles activate body's energy and bring about the cure. The very purpose of both these pathies is to arouse immense invisible physical and mental energy in the body by pressing various reflex points or by pricking acupuncture points so as to restore health and to keep the body in perfect order. Both these systems are based on holistic healing approach. "Holistic" is a term derived from Greek word, "holos" conveying the sense "whole", aiming at treating the patient as complete and undivided entity, incorporating three basic, characteristics of an individual- the body, the mind and the spirit. When treated collectively, the results are effective.

Neuro Acu -A System for All:

Neuro-Acu is a marvelous system, simple to understand and easy to practice, It is highly effective, completely safe and absolutely scientific. Whereas, acupuncture can only be carried out by a qualified and trained doctor, anybody educated or involved with other holistic therapies can benefit from Neuro Acu Therapy by understanding the theory of ten invisible zones in the body, location of various reflex points in hand, feet and other parts of the body and the technique of applying the pressure on these points. The best thing being Neuro Acu treatment can be given to people of any age men, women and babies, children, young and old anywhere and anytime. There is nothing to lose but too much to gain from this technique of therapy. Because of its unique qualities a large number of medical specialists having progressive and unbiased approach, speaks highly of this therapy.

Neuro Acu Theory-The Pivot of Acupressure

The concept of Neuro Acu therapy is the basis of reflexology or acupressure got new dimensions and scientific recognition when a distinguished American ENT specialist, Dr. William H. Fitzgerald undertook research during the early years of twentieth century to establish its practicality. His colleagues in the medical profession highly discouraged him, but his continuous research and dedicated efforts brought to light the presence of 10 energy zones in the body. These zones are in fact the basis of reflexology and acupressure.

Neuro Acu Therapy is very simple to understand. According to it there are ten invisible life force currents passing through the body from head to feet and palms in line with all the toes and fingers ending in the tips. The specific area falling under each life force current is called Zone (Neuro Acu). There are five longitudinal zones on right side of the body and five longitudinal on the left side of the body in equal proportions. All the ten zones run parallel over the entire body covering head, face, shoulder, arms hands, chest abdomen, reproductive organs, legs and feet.

Zone-1 Extends from top of the head to big toes in feet passing through the mid of forehead, nose, palate, lips, chin, chest, spine, abdomen and legs. Thus zone also goes up to thumbs covering shoulders and arms. Zone 1 thus feeds a part or entire area of the organs falling in this zone according to their actual position in the body namely head, brain, spine, nose mouth, chin, pituitary, pineal, thyroid, thymus and adrenal glands, lungs, heart (on the left as well as on right side), esophagus, stomach, duodenum, small intestine, liver (on right side), uterus, sex organs, prostate, urinary bladder, rectum and anus.

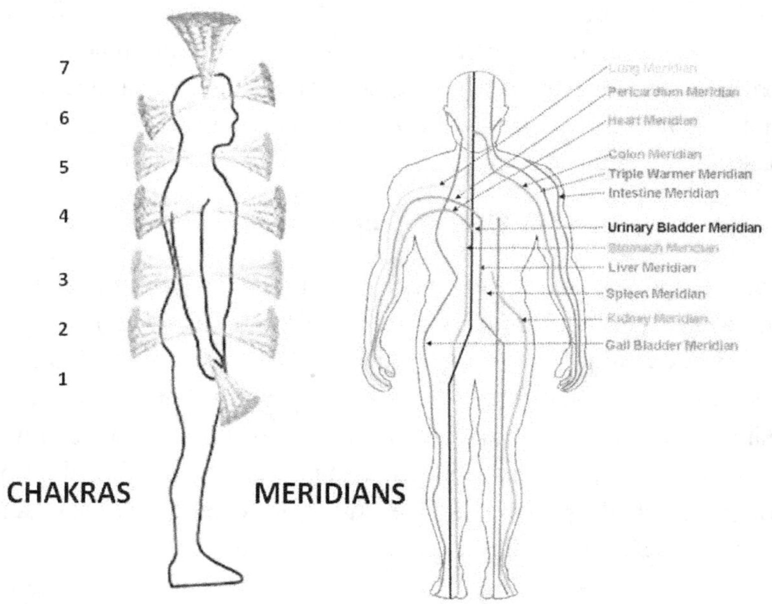

Division of body into longitudinal zones.

Zone-2 Comes from the top of the head and runs down to the second toe and likewise up to the tips of first finger. This zone covers certain portion of the brain, eyes, sinuses, tonsils, lungs, bronchial tubes, heart (on right and left, both sides), stomach, liver (on right side), solar plexus, pancreas (on left side), kidneys and small intestine.

Zone -3 Emanates from the top of the head and goes up to third toe in feet and also up to second finger in hands. It includes some portion of the brain, eyes, lungs, heart (on left side), stomach (on left side), solar plexus, pancreas (on left side), liver (on right side), kidneys, and appendix on right side and small intestine on both sides of the body.

Zone-4 Extends from top of the head down to fourth toe in feet and third finger in hands. This zone feeds certain area in brain, ears, shoulders, lungs, heart (on left side), stomach, spleen and pancreas (all three on the left side), liver, gall bladder and appendix (all three on right sides), small intestine and colon on both sides.

Zone-5 Moves from top of the head down to little toes and little fingers in the feet and hands, respectively. The fifth zone covers the outer side of the head, certain portion of the brain, ears, shoulders, upper arms, spleen (on left side), liver, gall bladder and appendix (all four on right side) and colon on both sides.

Although all the toes, thumbs and fingers embody reflex areas for the brain and head, but the major reflexes of the brain and head exist in big toe and thumbs. Interestingly, each big toe and thumb contains reflexes for half portion of brain and head on respective side. In addition each big toe and thumb sub divided into five zones.

From above it is clear that according to zone therapy, each foot and hand contains the reflex points of various organs falling in half portion of the body on that side as is evidence from the picture. To facilitate the quick and accurate detection of various Neuro Acu points pertaining to different organs, the founder of zone therapy has further divided hands and feet into transverse (horizontal) zones.

To get the desired results from the Neuro Acu therapy, it is imperative that one must possess the basic knowledge of the position of various organs in the body. A number of drawings inserted in this manual which gives the approximate location of the organs in the body and their reflex points in hand and feet.

Representation of Various Organs in Hands & Feet.

Part of Hand/Feet	Reflex Points of Organ
Big Toes/Thumbs	Head, Neck
Small Toes/Fingers	Head
Shoulder line to diaphragms line in feet/hands	Chest, lungs, shoulder
Arch (Upper Portion)	Diaphragm to waist portion of the body and the organs falling in upper abdominal area.
Heal	Pelvic area and sciatica nerve.
Inner foot/hand	Half portion of spine on right side and half portion on left side
Outer area of foot/hand	Arm, Shoulder, hip, leg, knee and lower back
Ankle area of feet/ wrists	Pelvic area, reproductive organs

Purpose:

The purpose of acupressure is to promote the body's own healing power, when key acupressure points on the surface of skin are pressed, muscular tension is released and the circulation of blood and body's vital life energy, (which Chinese call Chi energy) is promoted. Acupressure can be used to treat numerous conditions: effects of daily stress, headache, neck and shoulder pain, aches, pains, allergies, menstrual difficulties, fatigue, anxiety, insomnia, digestive problems, nausea, impotence and back pain etc.

Precautions:

Acupressure should not be used for certain conditions that require medical care such as serious burns, ulcer or infections, caution should be taken with the use of abdominal pressure points, especially when the patient has a life threating illness such as intestinal cancer or is pregnant.

Description:

Acupressure uses pressure usually applied with thumb, fingers, elbow, Knee or acupressure devices called Jimmy. The blockage of energy along these meridians can cause physical discomfort, pain, tension and stress.

The stimulation of points removes blockage by releasing muscle tension and allowing blood to flow more freely. It can also free an emotional blockage by releasing accumulated tension. The pressure may also release lactic acid that accumulates in muscles during vigorous exercise and is also removed from blood by the liver. It can however accumulate in muscles.

Light to medium pressure is applied to an acupressure point and it is to be rotated in a tight circle. In starting it is done with fingers, thumbs, hands, sometimes the elbows, knees are used for key pressure points. Since the more reactive points are tender or sensitive when pressed, this helps to determine the right location. If the response cannot be felt, the pressure points location may not be correct or pressure may not be strong enough. The sensation felt during acupressure treatment should be somewhere between pleasure and pain.

Three Benefits of Acupressure:

- **Diagnosis:** Instant and proper diagnose without a medical check up
- **Cure:** Cure of all types of diseases including that of cancer/brain and even HIV
- **Prevention:** Helps to prevent all types of diseases including heart problem, paralysis and even cancer.

Risks:

- There is no risk. Acupressure can be used with any other therapy. But it should not be replaced in lieu of other treatments/therapy.

A.B.C.... of Acupressure:

- A. Acupressure is great boon given to mankind by creator/Nature.

- B. Baby, just one day old can take treatment of acupressure.

- C. Cancer can be prevented, diagnosed and cured at Acupressure.

- D. Diagnosis made with acupressure is equal to MRI test can be done by oneself and without any much cost.

- E. Even a child of 10 years old can practice.

- F. Freedom from fears about all types of diseases, even cancer and AID/HIV.

How to apply Pressure:

Methods of applying pressure with Thumb.

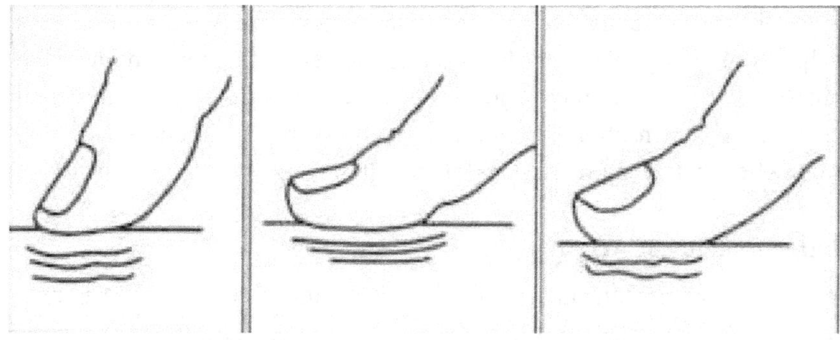

Correct technique of pressure application

Pointed finger or thumb, incorrect pressure technique

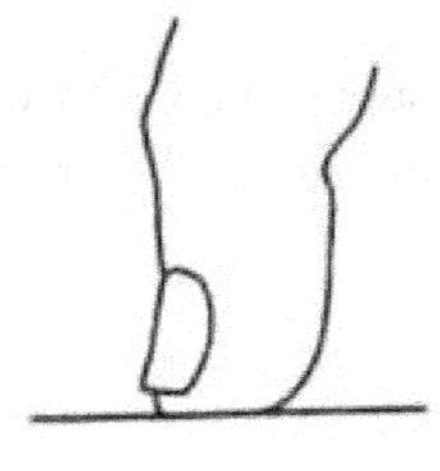

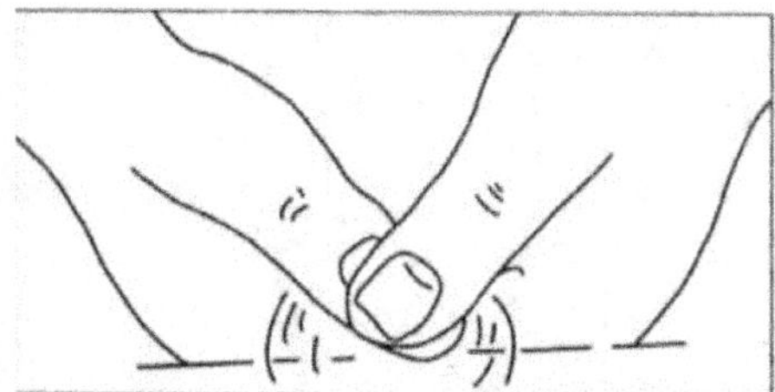

Thumbs of both hands can be used simultaneously to give effective pressure

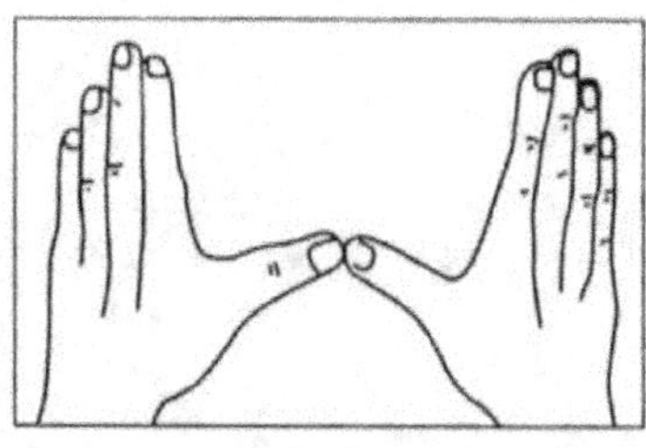

On the spine at special areas apply pressure with both thumbs

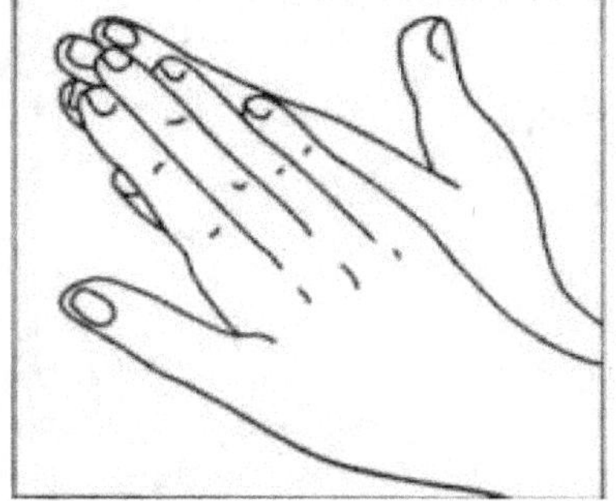

Apply pressure on some points like stomach with both hands at one time with three fingers together

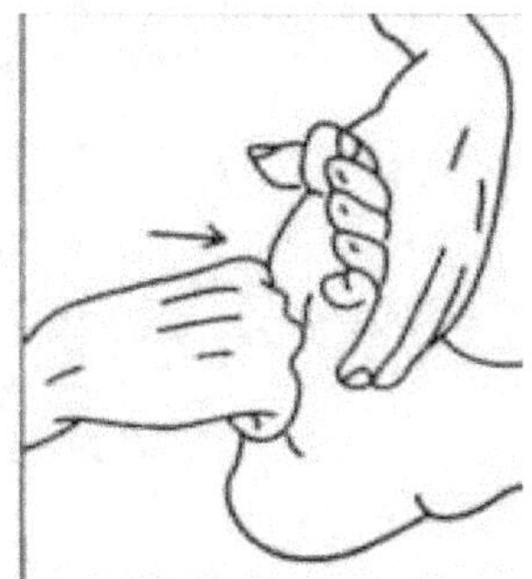

Apply pressure With knuckles at the sole of the feet

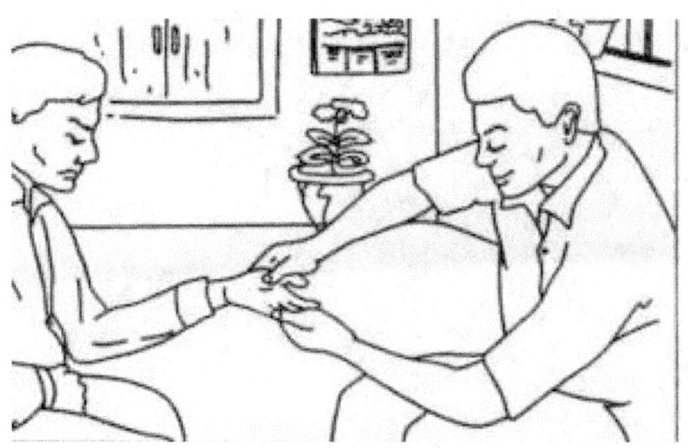

Methods of applying pressure on palm of the patient

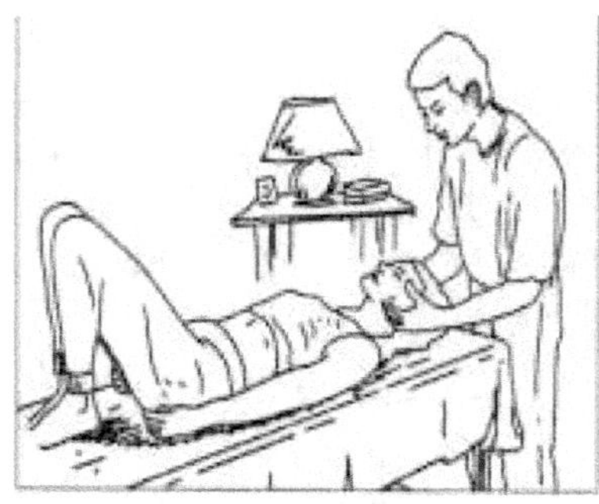

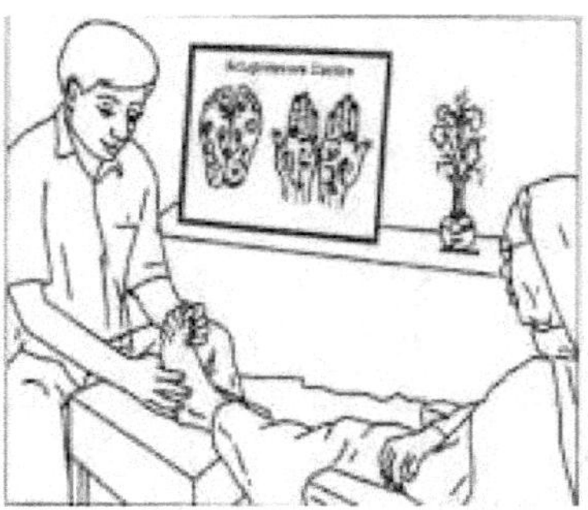

| Methods of applying pressure on the temple of the patient. | Methods of applying pressure sole of the foot of the patient |

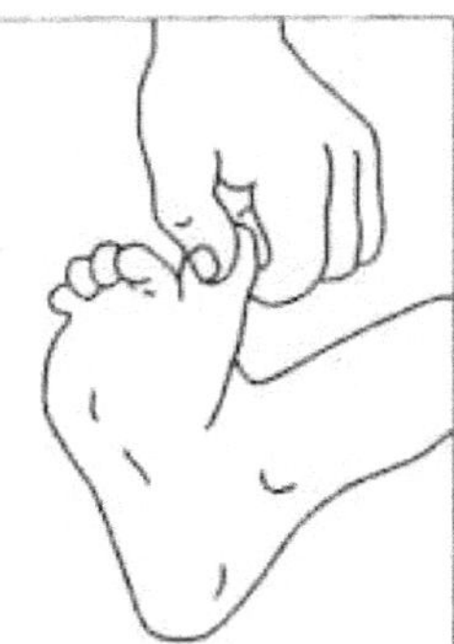

Techniques of application of pressure on the points concerning nervous system, especially the brain, lymphatic system, circulation and kidney must be pressed as these release tension and purge the body of harmful substances.

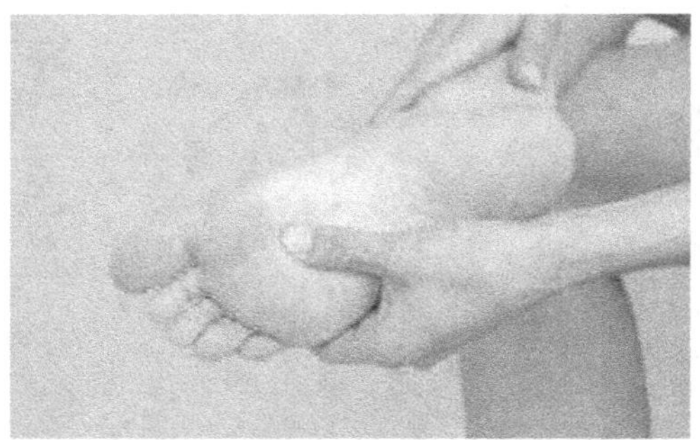

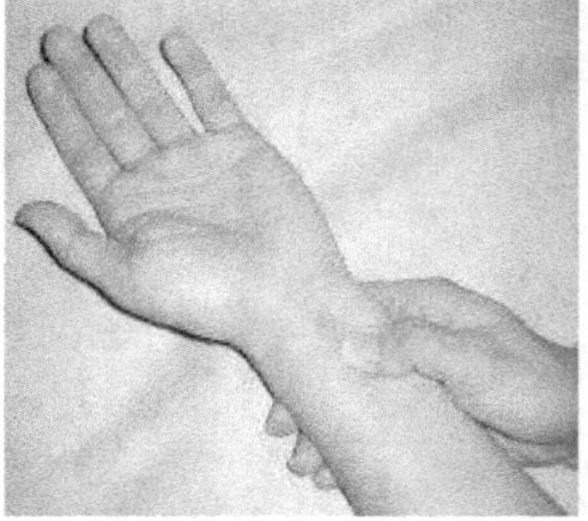

You can give pressure yourself without taking help of any one. Sit easy on chair, bed, and sofa or on floor as convenient

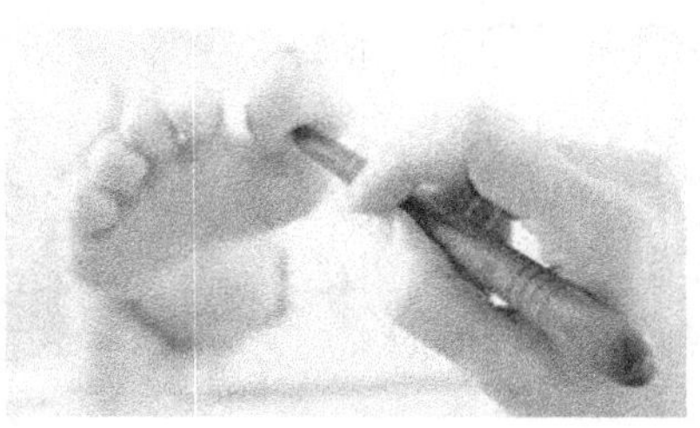 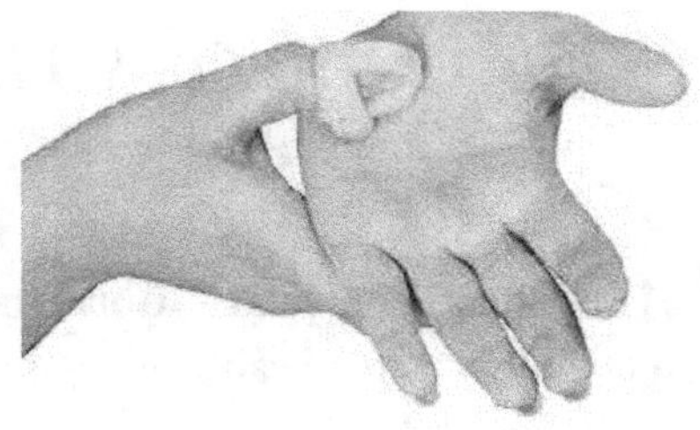

Way to give pressure on feet sole with Thumb/Jimmy to diagnose and treatment.

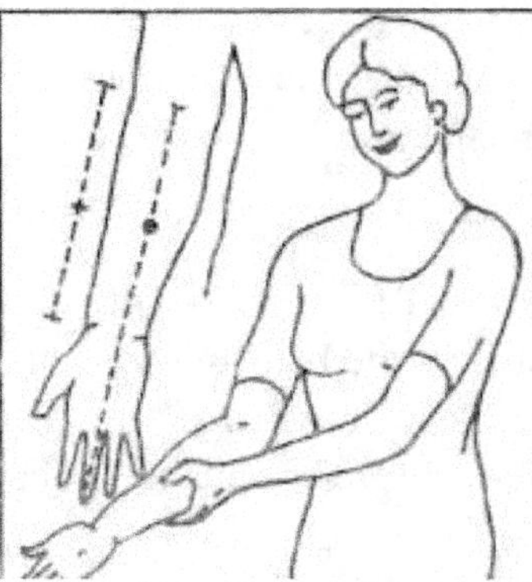

In the middle of right arm press this point three times in a tight circle morning and evening helps delay old age and keeps you youthful

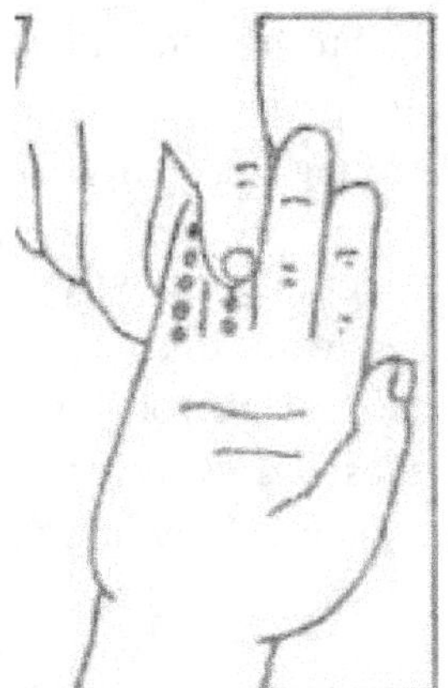

Any person if fall unconscious press these two fingers for couple of minutes on both hands the person will be normal very soon, and then give him/her some water to drink and make him/her lie for some time.

CODE OF ETHICS FOR THE PRACTITIONER

4.01. Social/Ecological Concern: Practitioners recognize their responsibility to the health and evolution of this planet.

4.02. Professional Conduct: Practitioner conduct themselves in a professional and ethical manner, perform only those services for which they are qualified, and represent their education, certification, professional affiliation and their qualifications honestly. They do not in any way profess to practice medicine or psychotherapy, unless licensed by their province.

4.03. Health History and Referrals: Practitioners keep accurate client records including profile of the body/mind health history. They discuss with clients any problem areas that may contraindicate use of acupressure techniques and refer clients to appropriate medical or psychological professionals when indicated.

4.04. Professional Appearance: Practitioners pay close attention to cleanliness, personal hygiene and professional appearance of self-clothing, of linens and equipment and of the office environment in general. They endeavor to provide a relaxing atmosphere, giving attention to reasonable scheduling and clarity about fees.

4.05. Communication and Confidentiality: Practitioners maintain clear and honest communications with their clients and keep all client information, whether medical or personal strictly confidential. They clearly disclose techniques used appropriately identifying each in the scope of their professional practice. They inform clients of legal limits to confidentiality.

4.06. Intention and Trust: Practitioners are encouraged to establish and maintain trust in the client relationship and to establish clear boundaries and atmosphere of safety.

4.07. Respect of Client: Practitioners respect the client's physical/emotional state and do not abuse clients through actions or words or silence, nor take advantage of therapeutic relationship. They in no way participate in sexual activities with a client. They consider the clients comfort zone for touch and for degree of pressure and the honor the client's requests a s much as possible within personal, professional and ethical limits. They acknowledge the inherent worth and individuality of each person and therefore do not unjustly discriminate against clients nor colleagues.

4.08. Professional Integrity: Practitioners represents restive organizations in a professional and compassionate manner. They represent themselves and their practice accurately and ethically. They conduct their business honestly. They do not give fraudulent information nor misrepresent themselves to students or clients. They do not act in a manner derogatory to the nature and positive intention of other professional organizations.

4.09. Professional Courtesy: Practitioners respect the standards set by Navkiran institute of holistic health sciences, respect service marks, trademarks and copyright laws. Professional courtesy includes respecting all ethical professionals in speech, writing or otherwise and communicating clearly with others.

4.10. Professional Excellence: Practitioners strive for professional excellence through regular assessment of personal and professional strengths and weaknesses, and by continued education and training.

IMPORTANT WARNINGS & INSTRUCTIONS

Warnings: - Don't use acupressure to replace standard emergency procedures or incensed medical treatment. If the person is seriously injured or have persistent symptoms seek urgent medical treatment.

Acupressure should not be used: -

- As the only treatment for the illness; if the condition is serious see a doctor.

- If the person have a heart condition

- Just before or within 20 minutes after heavy exercise, a large meal, or bathing.

- If the point in question under a mole, wart, varicose vein, abrasion, bruise, cut or any other break in the skin.

- If pregnant especially if more than 3 months.

Acupressure is not appropriate as the only treatment for acute or chronic conditions. If needed, seek medical attention or emergency help. Some symptoms and conditions include cautions and warnings. For these symptoms, only use acupressure to supplement professional medical care, or when no professional medical care is available. Only try acupressure for these symptoms **after** seeking professional care and after using standard first aid and emergency techniques.

Directions for Using Acupressure

To stimulate an acupoint properly, you must apply deep probing pressure. Therefore, only apply pressure with:

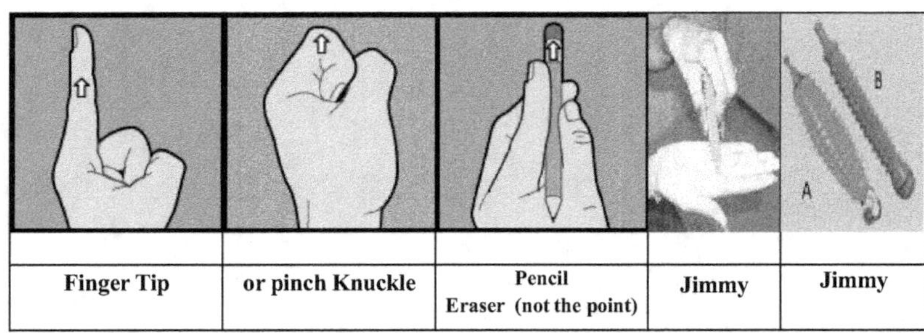

Finger Tip	or pinch Knuckle	Pencil Eraser (not the point)	Jimmy	Jimmy

HOW TO DIAGNOSE

Qualification

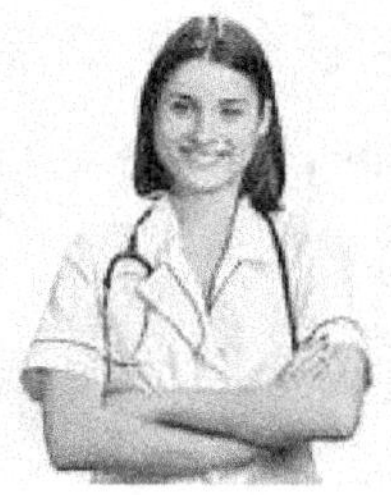

First and foremost qualification of Holistic Healer or Acupressure Therapist is his/her own fitness and health. Not only body but also mind. One should be cheerful and free from any prejudice. The practitioner should be following the same therapy for himself and family members for which you will be preaching for others. You must remember that the patient is a human being and has come to get rid of his/her problems and clear doubts about his ailments.

First Clue:

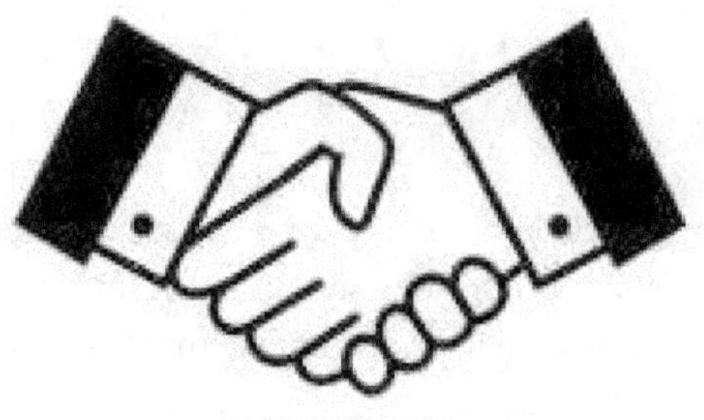

A warm smile and welcoming handshake is what a patient expects. When you shake hand with the patient, you get a clue about the problem. If the patient is younger than yourself- his/her palm should be warmer than yours. However, if the palm is cooler, you will know that the energy flow in the patient's body is less. Similarly, if the patient is older than you, the palm should be cooler. But if the palm is warmer, it indicates that there is excess heat in the body or the patient has fever.

Solar Plexus: Solar plexus controls Äpan Vayu" and so regulates the movements of stools and urine; also controls all organs below the diaphragm.

Methods to confirm the solar plexus is in order or not

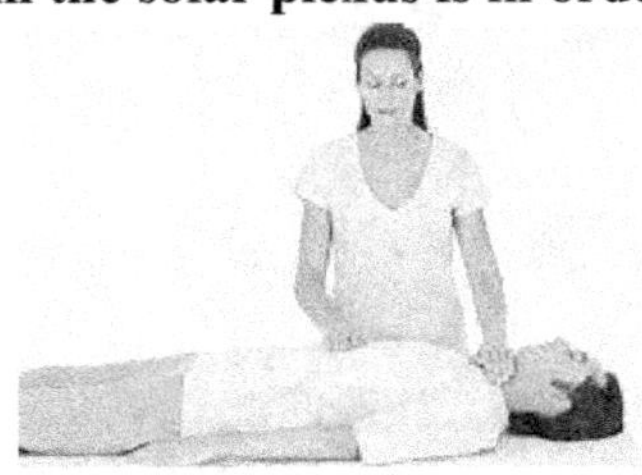

In the morning, on an empty stomach, when you lie down on any hard surface on your back and if you press your finger or thumb in the navel, you will feel a throbbing sound just like the thumping of heart, it means that the system is perfectly fine.

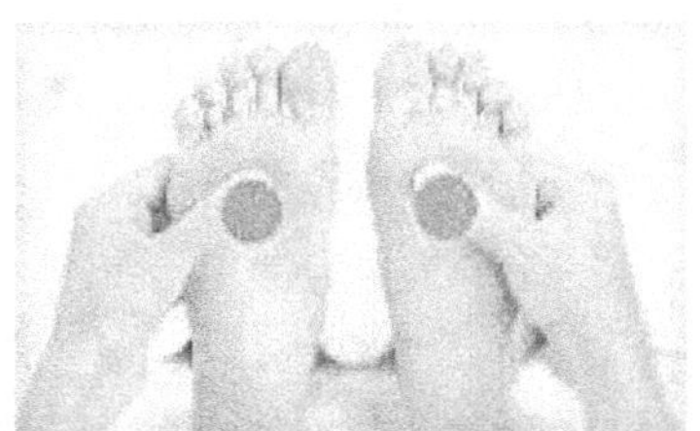

Lie down on your back, arms straight by your sides, keep legs straight and toes upright. The two big toes should be in level with each other as shown in the pic below, if they are not, it indicates the disturbance of Solar Plexus.

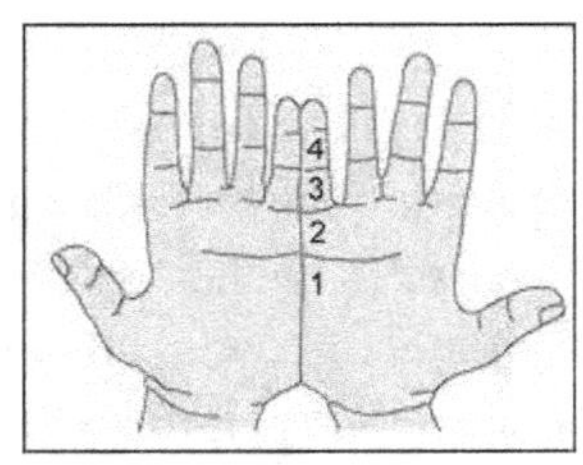

Join the two palms and match the lines 1and 4 as shown in the picture below. These lines will match with each other. If the solar plexus is in order. If the solar plexus has shifted line No. 4 will not match.

To set Solar Plexus in order:

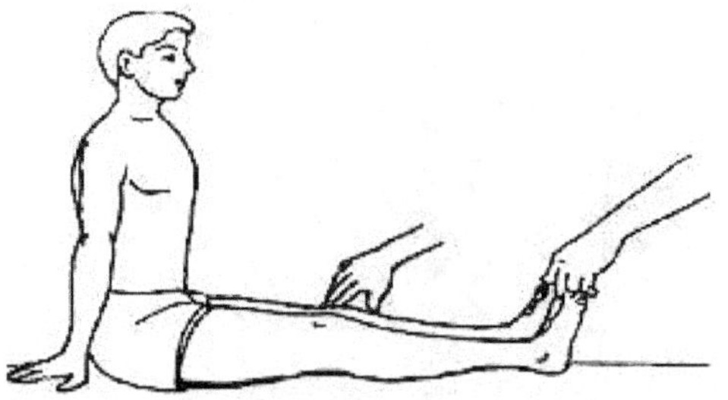

Solar Plexus Correction (Big Toe Method)-Or Lay on flat surface

Correct the solar plexus by pressing with one hand and knee of the leg whose big toe is lower and keep the middle finger of the other hand in between the two big toes and holding them, pull up only the big toe which is lower. After 2-3 pull ups check the level of two big toes. If the level has not come in line, repeat the procedure till the level is proper. Only in a few rare cases, where there is a natural difference in the feet of the patient, this method will not work.

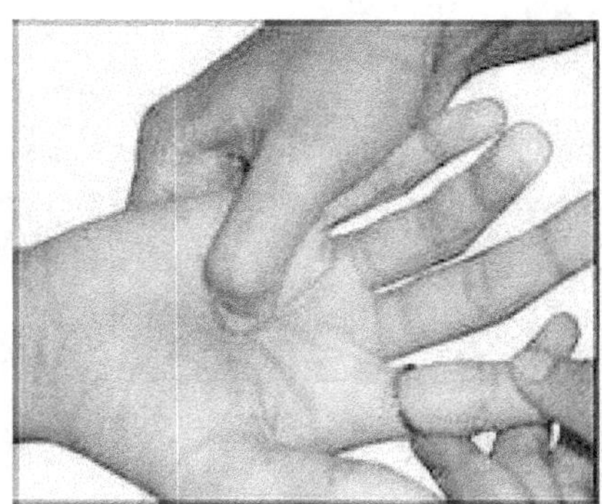
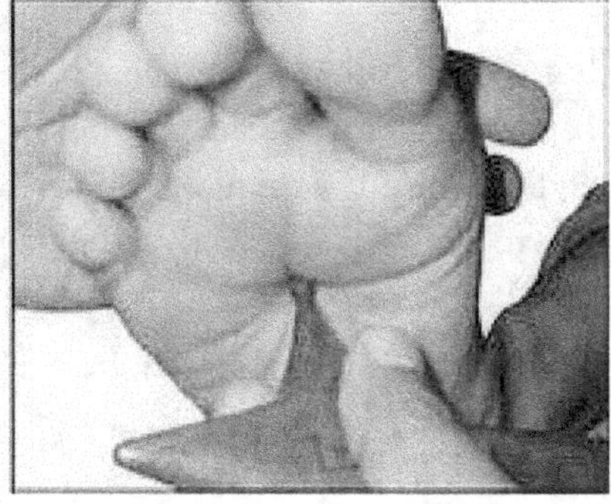

Look at hand and feet chart and give pressure on point No 29. Press points of solar plexus intermittently in both the palms not only from the

front side but also from back of the hands. After half a minute verify whether the solar plexus has come in order.

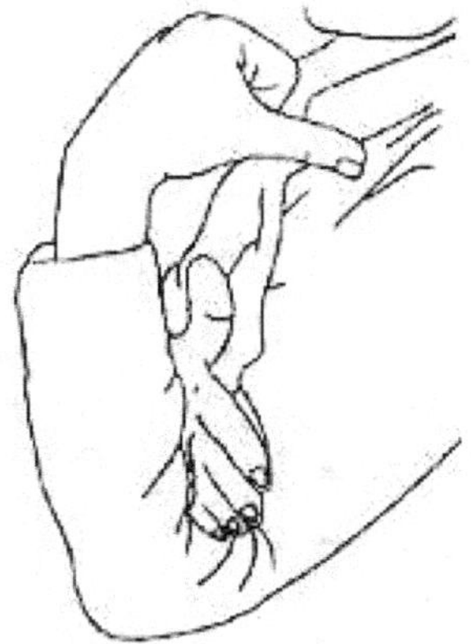

Solar Plexus Correct - Elbow Method

Keep your right palm vertically on the joint of elbow of the left hand and try to touch the left shoulder with the thumb with a jerk. Repeat five times. In the same way do with the right hand and then join both palms and match the lines 1 to 4 to verify whether the solar plexus is in order or not.

This method is the easiest way to correct the solar plexus. It is advisable to do this exercise every morning, whether the solar plexus is in order or not.

Put a small oil lamp/candle on the Navel (A coin or some else can be kept on navel as a base to hold the candle), cover it with a metal glass and press it for a minute. The air inside will burn out and a vacuum will be created. This vacuum will bring the solar plexus to the center. Then lift glass from one side after one minute. Repeat it for three to four times

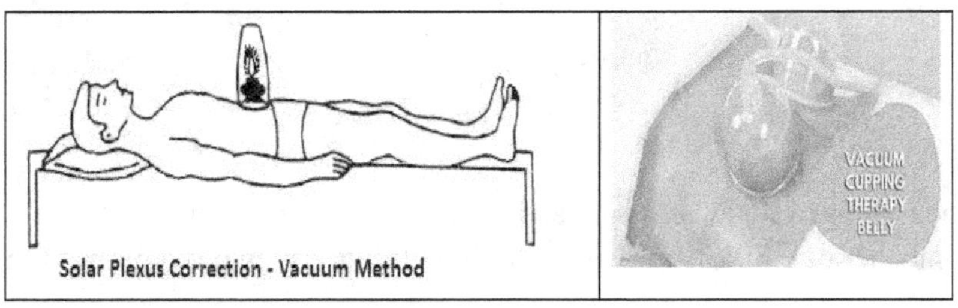

Solar Plexus Correction - Vacuum Method

till the throbbing is felt at the center. After correcting solar plexus, drink warm water or green tea or ginger tea.

In case of chronic problem like diarrhea, vomiting, stomach upset etc. The solar plexus may shift up or down and will be necessary to correct it at least two to three times in a day.

Even a minor difference in the level of big toes indicates that solar plexus is not in order. It may be noted that upward shifting of solar plexus leads to constipation and if it becomes chronic, this can lead to piles and even colon cancer too. The muscles above the navel become stiff and this problem is many times termed as Hiatus Hernia.

Similarly when the solar plexus has shifted downwards it leads to loose motion. This often is wrongly diagnosed as diarrhea and the prescribed treatment ends up by damaging the whole digestive system. The drugs taken to control such diarrhea can leads to acidity and ulcer and long term diarrhea leads to colic pain, anemia and serious consequences like cancer.

In the case of children too, the correction of solar plexus is very important. For a breast feed baby if the mother has gastric problem, the baby's solar plexus also gets damaged either leading to constipation or loose motion.

What should be done in case of frequent shifting of the solar plexus: - Due to frequent gas trouble, weakness of intestine, lifting of heavy articles, sometimes there is a shifting of the solar plexus. In case of such frequent shifting of solar plexus following treatment should be followed:

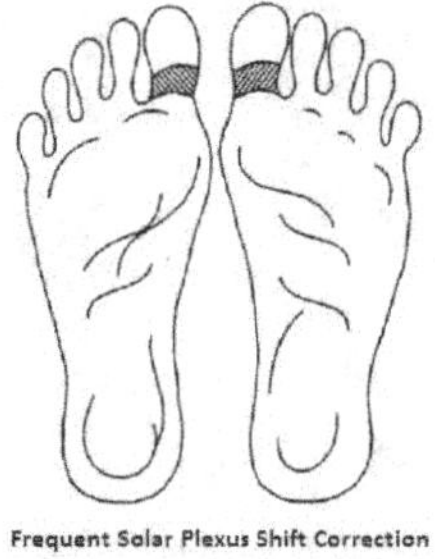

Frequent Solar Plexus Shift Correction

First correct the solar plexus. Take little string (Thicker than the sewing thread) and tie eight to nine rounds of this thread around the base of the big toe. It should not be very tight, then make a knot (as shown in the pic) do the same with the other toe and ask the patient to keep it minimum for 3 days. During this period, this thread can be removed if there is unbearable pain in the big toe.

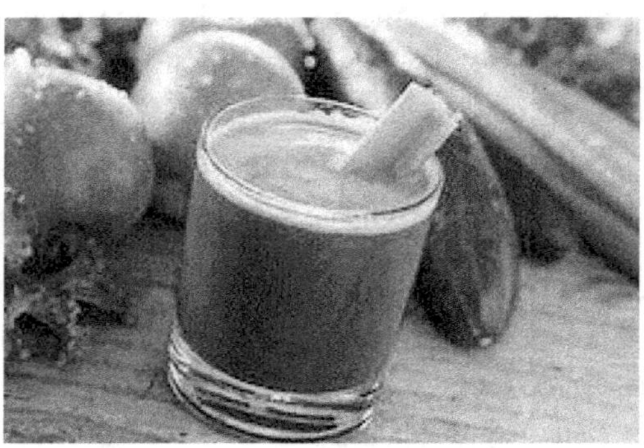

For complete cure patient should have a diet of green juice, fruit juices and light foods and also do some exercise or yoga to strengthen the muscles of the digestive system.

Eyes: -Similarly, the eyes reveal the vitality of the body, in case of a healthy person; the eyes would be shining radiating health and happiness.	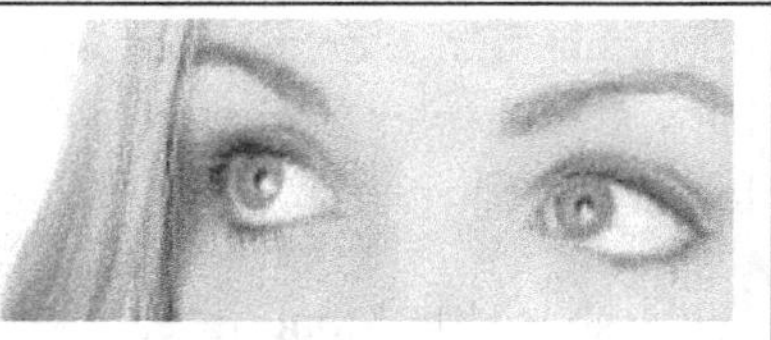
If the eyes of the patient are whitish and there is no redness in the corners of the eyes, it denotes anemic conditions, which could be due to worms and so you should press the middle of outside part of nails of small finger/toes. And if you observe pain on that point, it indicates that there are worms in the intestine of the patient.	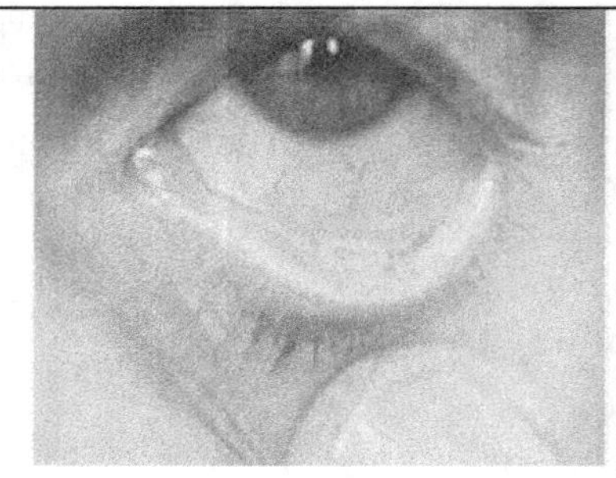

Then carefully observe the eyes if there are dark circles and swelling below them, it denotes that kidney of the patient are not functioning properly and so you should check up point **No.26** of the kidney in both palms and sole of the feet (as shown in the pic below)

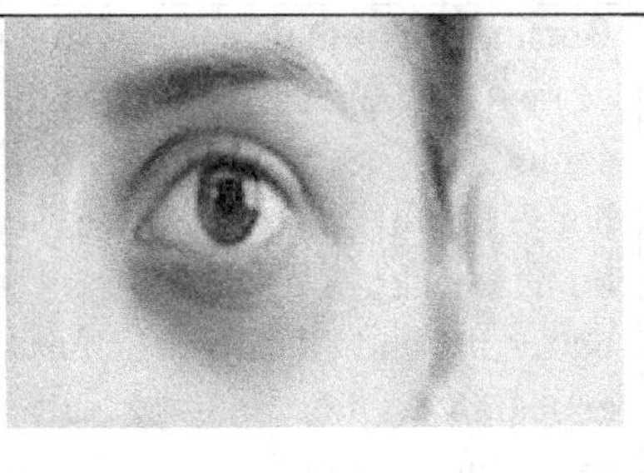

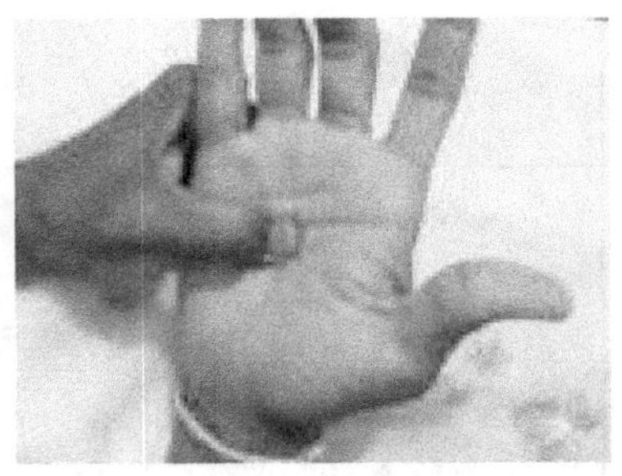

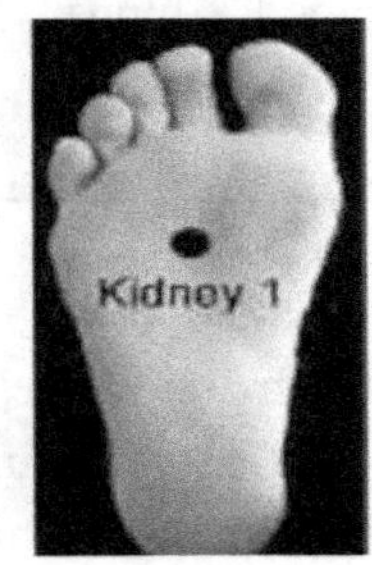

Face: Your face is a road map of your health, like your eyes are the windows to your soul. While emotions get reflected on your face, the different parts of your face reveal the status of your health.

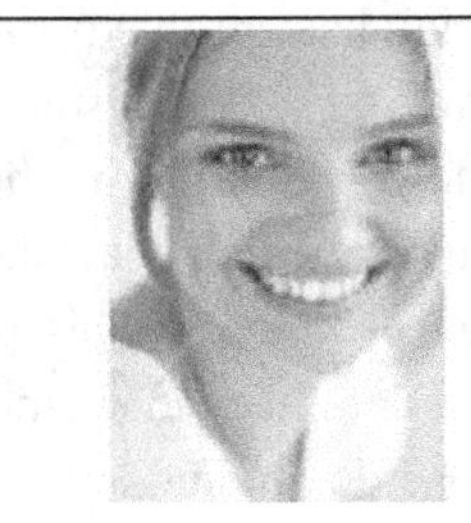

Yellowing of Skin and Eyes: -If you notice a yellow tinge around your face and specifically the whites of your eyes turning yellow, it is a big sign that you may be suffering from jaundice.

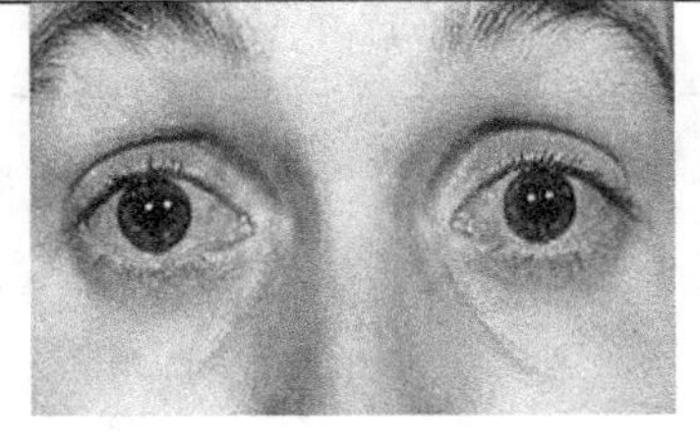

Butterfly-Shaped Rash: -Any kind of rash on the face is a sure sign that something is wrong within your body. If the rash stretches across both cheeks in the shape of a butterfly and has a sunburn-like appearance, you may be suffering from lupus. Lupus is an immune-system disorder that affects the skin, joints, blood, lungs, heart and kidneys.

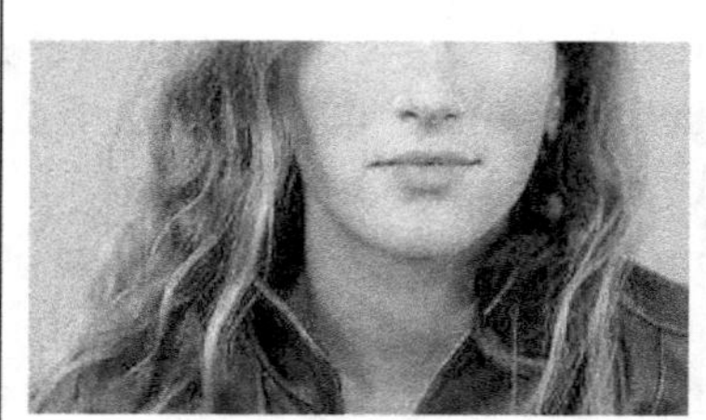

Excessive Facial Hair: - Unwanted hair along the jaw line, chin and upper lip can be very embarrassing for any woman. This beauty problem is known as hirsutism.

This facial hair problem can be a symptom of polycystic ovary syndrome (PCOS), a hormone imbalance in which male hormone levels are elevated. This problem is more common in women after menopause due to sudden hormonal changes in the body.

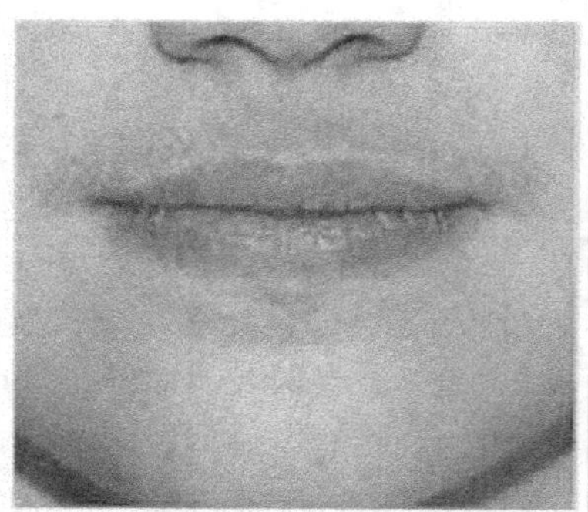

Pale Skin: -If person is otherwise healthy looking skin suddenly appears pale, washed-out and lifeless, get your iron level checked. Iron- deficiency anemia, which affects billions of people worldwide, is one of the main causes of pale-looking skin. Due to a low iron level, the body cannot produce sufficient hemo- globin, which is needed to give your blood its red color and your skin its healthy tone.

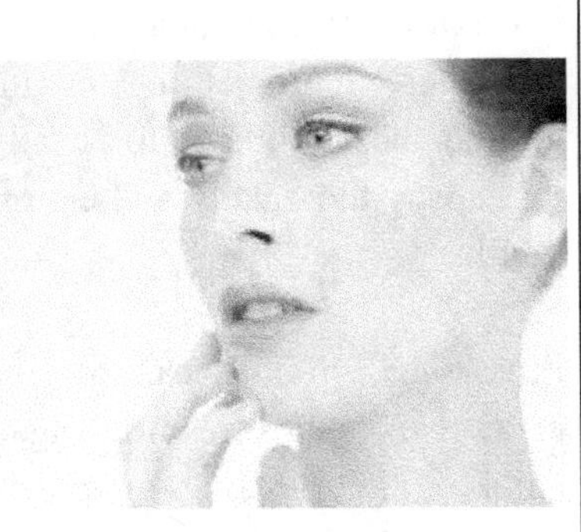

Dry Skin and Flaky Lips: - Everyone experiences dry skin from time to time. It can be due to minor causes, such as wintry air or overly hot showers. However, at times, excessive dry skin as well as flaky and chapped lips is a classic sign of dehydration.

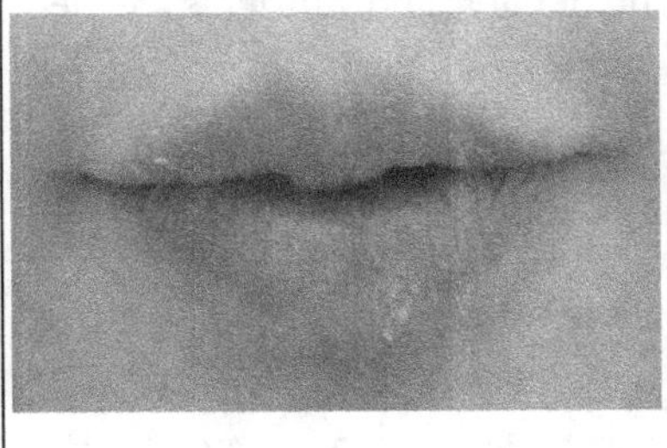

Abnormal Skin Discoloration: - Women who have PCOS may notice thick, brown or black patches on the neck folds, forehead, navel, armpits and breasts. This type of skin discoloration is known as acanthosis nigricans. Insulin resistance or high insulin levels in people suffering from PCOS causes the appearance of thick, corrosive and discolored skin on various parts of the body.

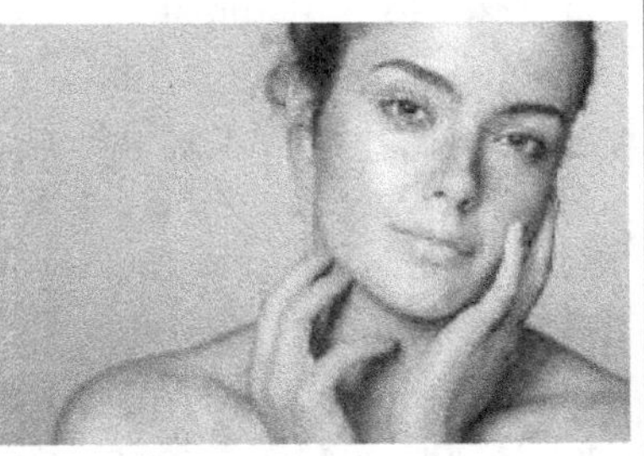

Deep Premature Wrinkles: - Wrinkles are inevitable with age. However, premature wrinkles around the mouth or forehead can take away the beauty and charm of youth.

Premature wrinkles can be due to excessive exposure to cigarette smoke. The nicotine in cigarettes narrows the blood vessels in the skin's outer layers and reduces blood flow. This deprives your skin of oxygen and nutrients needed for healthy and beautiful skin.

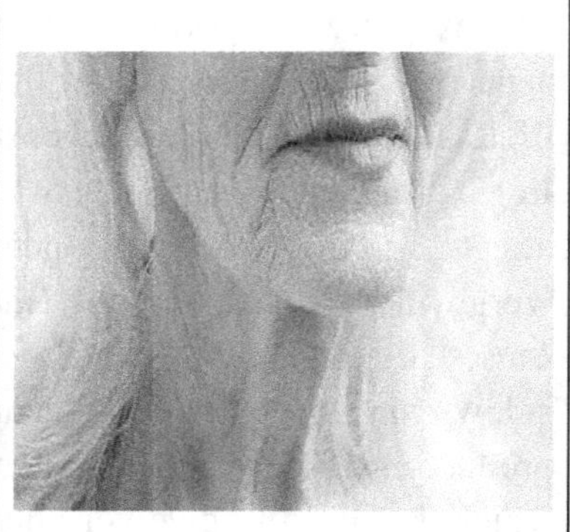

Cracks at the Corners of the Mouth:- Cracks near the mouth, which are medically known as angular cheilitis, are often associated with vitamin B2 or riboflavin deficiency.
Lack of this B vitamin in the body can lead to inflammation of the membranes of your mouth, skin, eyes and gastrointestinal tract. Along with cracks at the corners of your mouth, you can also suffer from symptoms like swelling of the mucous membranes, inflamed eyelids, sores on your lips or mouth, and skin redness.

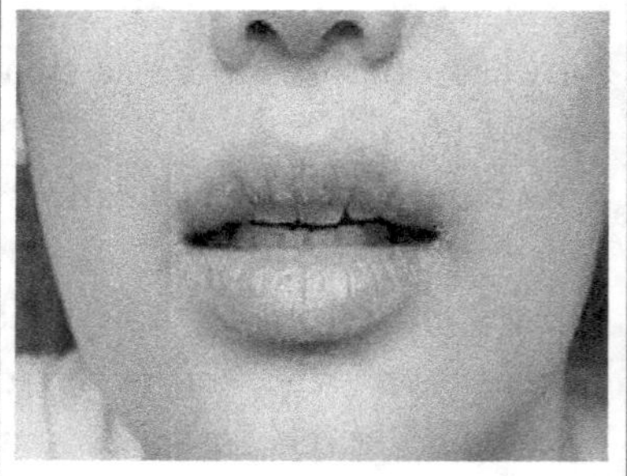

Yellow Patches around the Eyes: - Yellow patches in the skin around the eyes, known as xanthelasma, can be a sign of heart disease. Xanthelasma palpebrarum are yellow plaques that occur most commonly near the inner canthus of the eyelids. These small skin patches are soft and painless and don't interfere with vision. However, this problem is often associated with atherosclerosis, dyslipidemia and coronary artery disease.

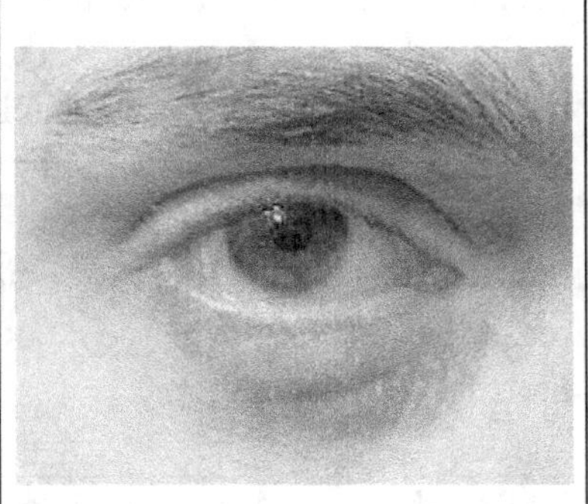

Puffy Eye: - Puffy eyes or dark circles under the eyes typically result from too many late nights or not getting enough sleep. It can even be due to too much crying. However, if puffy eyes occur more often despite getting enough sleep, it may signal an underlying medical problem.

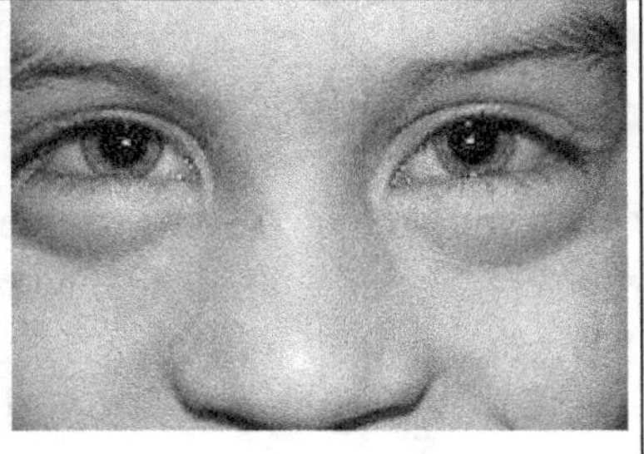

Black Pigments: -If you observe black pigmentation mixing with the original skin color of the face, it could be due to excess heat in the body or some skin problem or even an indication of HIV.

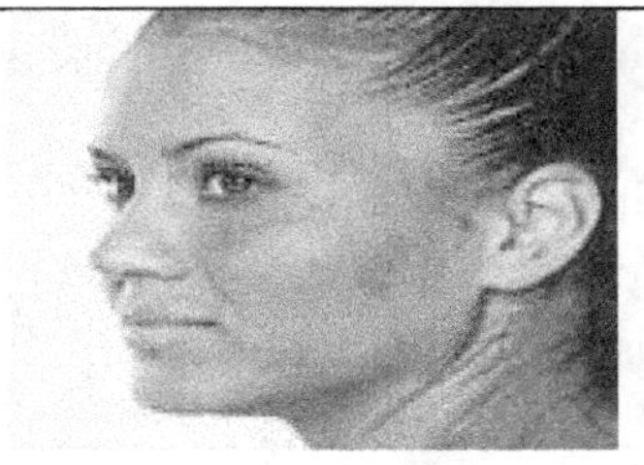

Males: - If you observe that the growth of the beard has not been all over the face and there are patches where the beards have not grown, then it indicates sex problem in males. It could be excessive masturbation and for that just check nails for the half –moons.

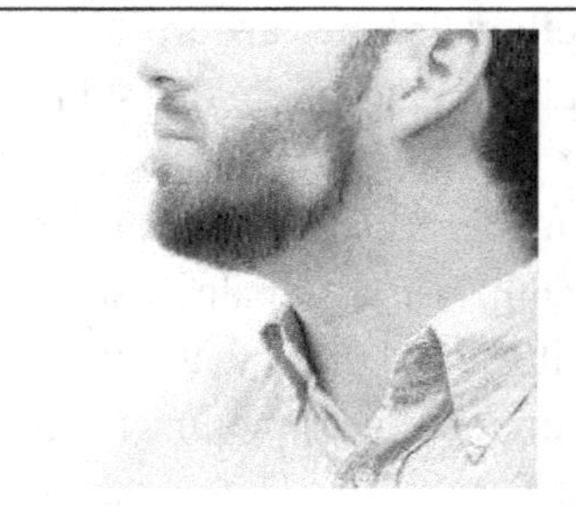

Nails: -Nails can reveal clues to your overall health; If the half-moons are milky white and so prominent that they look as though they are pasted on the nails and sparkling, new light comes in the eyes reflecting virile, vibrant health. These youngsters look attractive and their manners become pleasant. The syndrome of the body becomes powerful and immune system becomes sound and strong enough to prevent any disease. It is like spring for the youth.

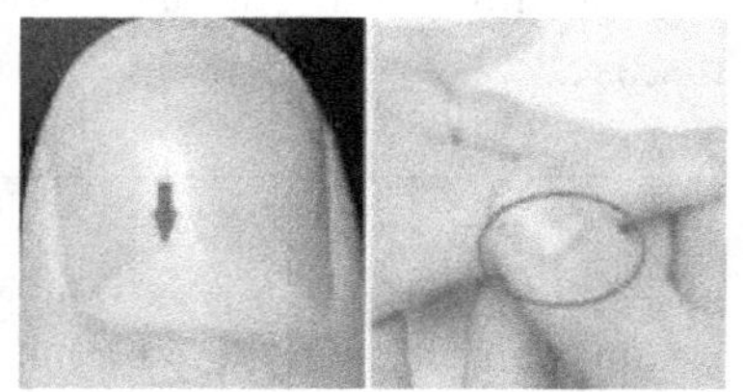

Pale Nails: - Very pale nails can sometimes be a sign of serious illness, such as: Anemia, Congestive heart failure, Liver disease, Malnutrition.

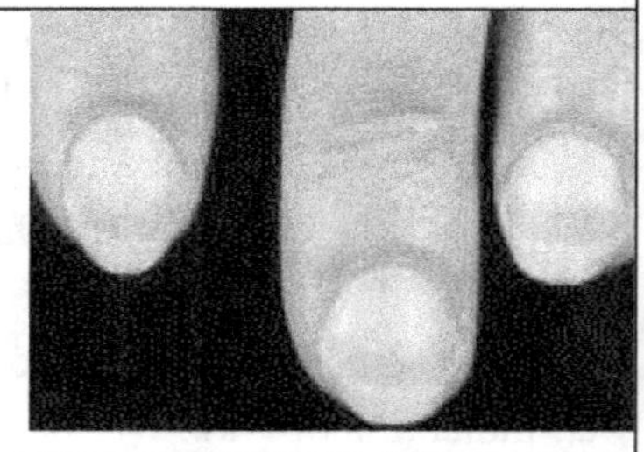

White Nails with darker Rims: - If the nails are mostly white with darker rims, this can indicate liver problems, such as hepatitis. In this image, you can see the fingers are also jaundiced, another sign of liver trouble.	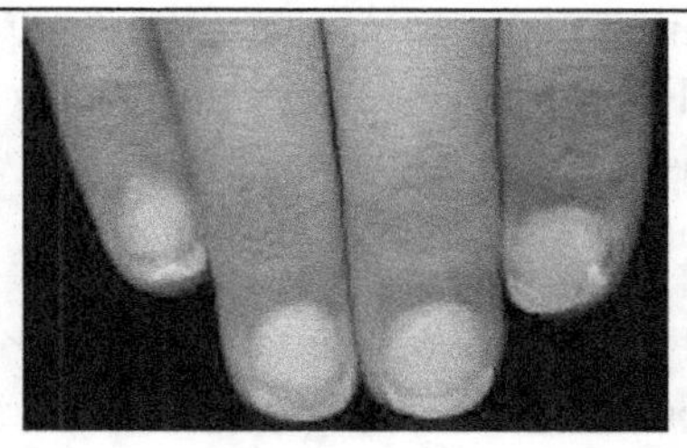
Yellow Nails: -One of the most common causes of yellow nails is a fungal infection. As the infection worsens, the nail bed may retract, and nails may thicken and crumble. In rare cases, yellow nails can indicate a more serious condition such jaundice.	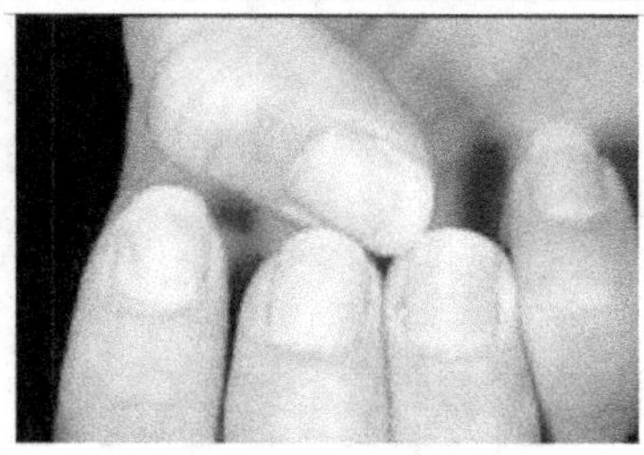
Cracked or Split Nails: -Dry, brittle nails that frequently crack or split has been linked to thyroid disease. Cracking or splitting combined with a yellowish hue is more likely due to a fungal infection.	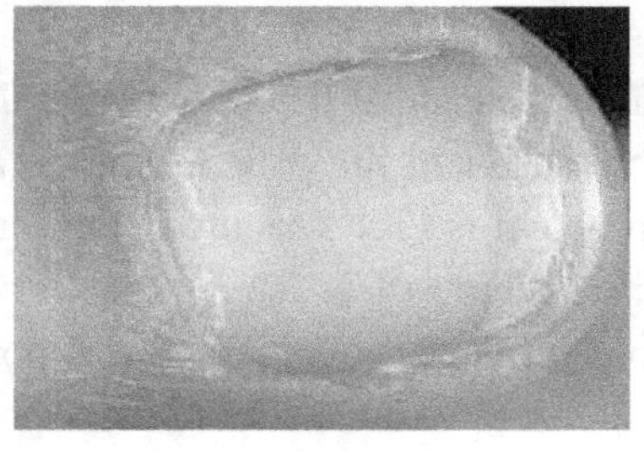

Barometer of the Body:

Next, checkup point no. 8 of the Thyroid/Parathyroid gland. This is the barometer of the body. In case of any complaint anywhere in the main functioning of organs of the body, for more than eight days there will be a hurting pain on this point when pressed. It is no surprise that its points on palms and soles are biggest which indicates its importance. In case there is no pain on these points, when pressed, it indicates that patient is healthy and the problem is minor and there is nothing to worry about it, and inform the patient accordingly. Many a times, the patient has a little doubt of having something wrong in his/her body. So when the patient is assured that there is nothing to worry about, he/she is relieved from unnecessary worry and tension.

The degree of pain on the point denotes the severity and extent of problem in the body. Such seriousness can be measured from the following illustration.

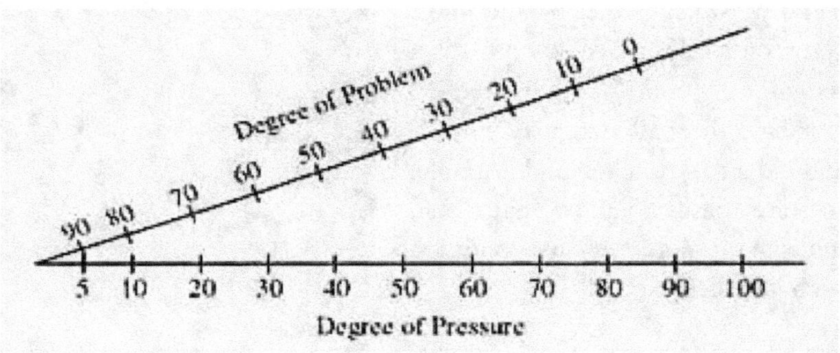

This means that when you press this point event slightly, i.e. 5 degree of pressure and the patient cries in agony, it denotes that degree wise the problem is very serious. In the same way, when you press very hard say 100 degree of pressure, and there is no pain or flicker in the eyes of patient, it denotes that there is no problem. From experience one would be able to know the exact degree of such seriousness.

Similarly, the degree if damage to any organ, can be found out by the above illustration chart, i.e. when pressed slightly on point no 6 of throat and if there is severe pain. It denotes inflamation of tonsils due to bacterial or viral infection, causing a sore throat, fever and difficulty in swallowing.

Even when a person thinks he is healthy and if there's some noticeable problem developing inside the body or maybe there are some slight symptoms which are generally neglected then pressure on point no. 8 will immediately reveal the internal problem of the body.

How to reach the root cause:-

After you have checked the solar plexus and corrected it. If necessary, press on point no 8 and when you find pain on the same, proceed further and ask patient his/her complaints and go on pressing on corresponding points. However, never come to any conclusion about diagnosis till you are satisfied about the root cause.

It's a fact that in India and other less advanced countries, patients are not willing to discuss their sex and menstrual problems. But Neuro Acupressure can lead you to the root cause. For proper diagnose, it's most important to study the following Neuro Acupressure Charts and about the functioning of all endocrine glands and lymph glands. (Lymph Glands Point No.16. although they are not endocrine glands because of their importance, they have been included here. The point of these glands is under Point No. 16 in the middle of wrists. They control the immune defence system of our body, prevents the formation of pus on any cut or boil on the body and quickly heals the wounds.

These glands help to clear the toxin from the body- clear the dead cells from the system. But when such toxins and dead cells are in excess, these glands have to over work and they becomes weak and tender. At that time, when you press on the point of these glands, it pains. If such pain continues, it means that these glands are not able to stop the malignant growth forming from toxins and dead cells. As such the first symptom to detect Cancer even at a very early stage is to find out whether there is any pain on this gland. Moreover, it has also been found that if there is a pain on these glands and also on the point of pancreas Point No.25, it indicates Diabetes, increase of glucose in the blood. Thus you will observe that to prevent Cancer and Sugar in the blood, it's most necessary to keep these glands in active condition. Further hurting on this Point No. 18 denotes possibility of HIV/AIDS.

Our body is really a great wonder. It reveals any small problem on these points of palms and soles. (It may be noted that the diagnosis made by Neuro Acupressure is so accurate that on several occasions, I have the privilege to challenge the diagnosis made with X ray and other medical tests.

PRESSURE POINTS

Point No.	Organ/Body Part	Point No.	Organ/Body Part
1.	Brain	20.	Colon
2.	Mental Nerve	21.	Appendix (Front) Allergy (Back)
3.	Pituitary	22.	Gallbladder
4.	Pineal	23.	Liver
5.	Head Nerves	24.	Shoulder
6.	Throat	25.	Pancreas
7.	Neck	26.	Kidney
8.	Thyroid/Parathyroid	27.	Stomach
9.	Spine	28.	Adrenal
10.	Piles	29.	Solar Plexus
11.	Prostrate	30.	Lungs
12.	Penis	31.	Ear
13.	Vagina	32.	Energy
14.	Uterus	33.	Nerves of Ear
15.	Testes/Ovaries	34.	Cold
16.	Lymph Gland (front side), Lower Lumbar (back of wris)	35. 36.	Eyes Heart
17.	Hip & Knee	37.	Spleen
18.	Bladder	38.	Thymus
19.	Intestine	39.	Optic Nerve

Left Hand

Sinus points
34 Cold
34 Cold
33 Ear & Nerve
32 Energy
Brain
Pituitary
Pineal
Mental nerves
3
4
2
5 Head nerves
Throat
6
7 Neck
35 Eye
35 Eye
31 Ear
31 Ear
30 & 38
Adrenal 28
Lungs
Thymus
Pancreas
29 S.P
25
36 Heart
24 — Shoulder
27 Stomach
26 Kidney
37 Spleen
8
Thyroid & Parathyroid
23 Colon
19 Intestines
18 Bladder
17 — Hip & Knee
Piles — 10
Prostate — 11
Penis — 12
Vagina — 13
16 Lymph glands
15 — Testes & Ovaries
14 — Uterus

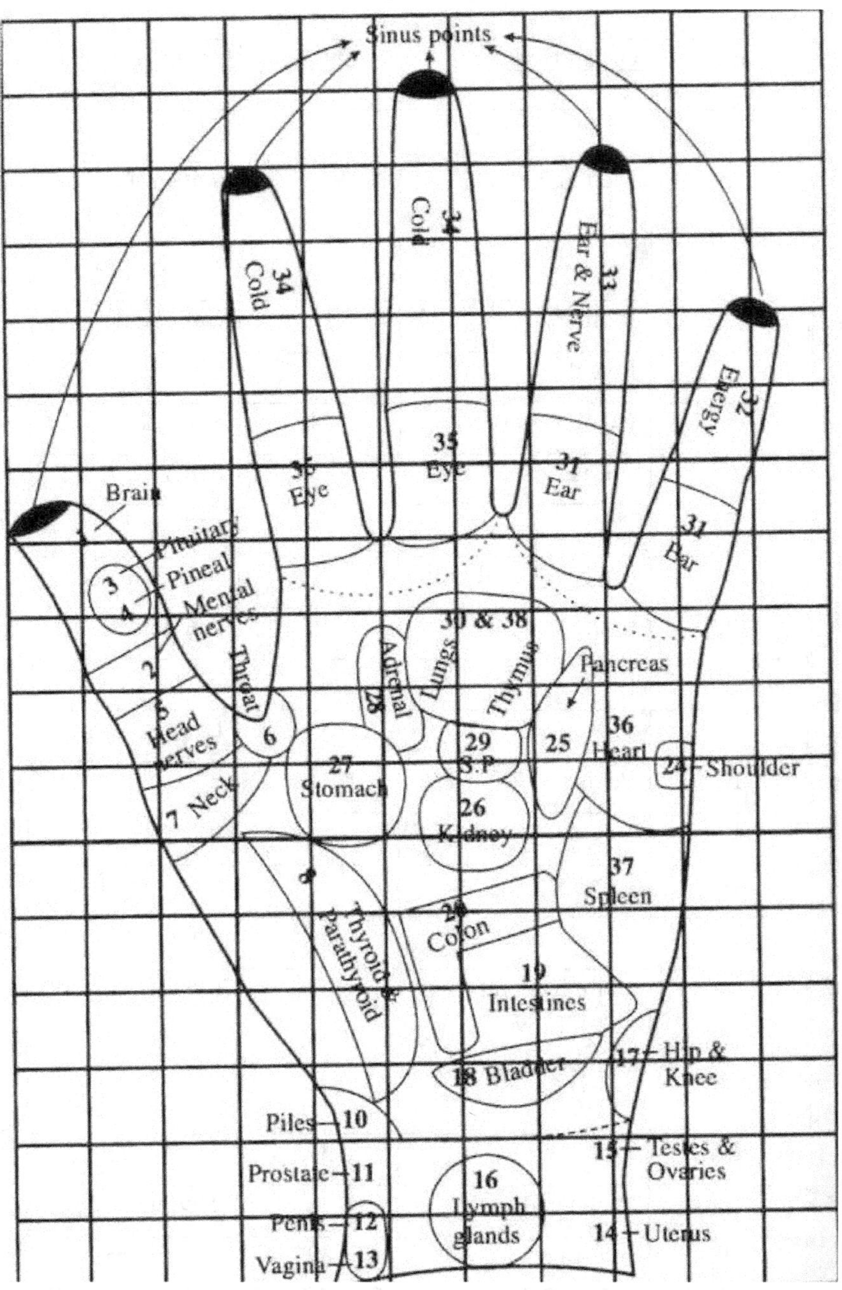

Right Hand

Sinus points
34 Cold
34 Cold
Ear-Nerve
33
32 Energy
31 Ear
31 Ear
35 Eye
35 Eye
1 Brain
3
4
Pituitary
Pineal
2
5
Mental Nerves
Head Nerves
Throat
30 & 38 Lungs Thymus
28 Adrenal
25 Pancreas
23
Shoulder 24
Liver
6
27 Stomach
29 S. P.
7 Neck
Gall Bladder 22
26 Kidney
20 Colon
8 Thyroid & Parathyroid
Appendix 21
19 Intestines
Hip & Knee 17
18 Bladder
Testes & Ovaries 15
10 Piles
16 Lymph glands
11 Prostate
Uterus 14
12 Penis
13 Vagina
Right Hand

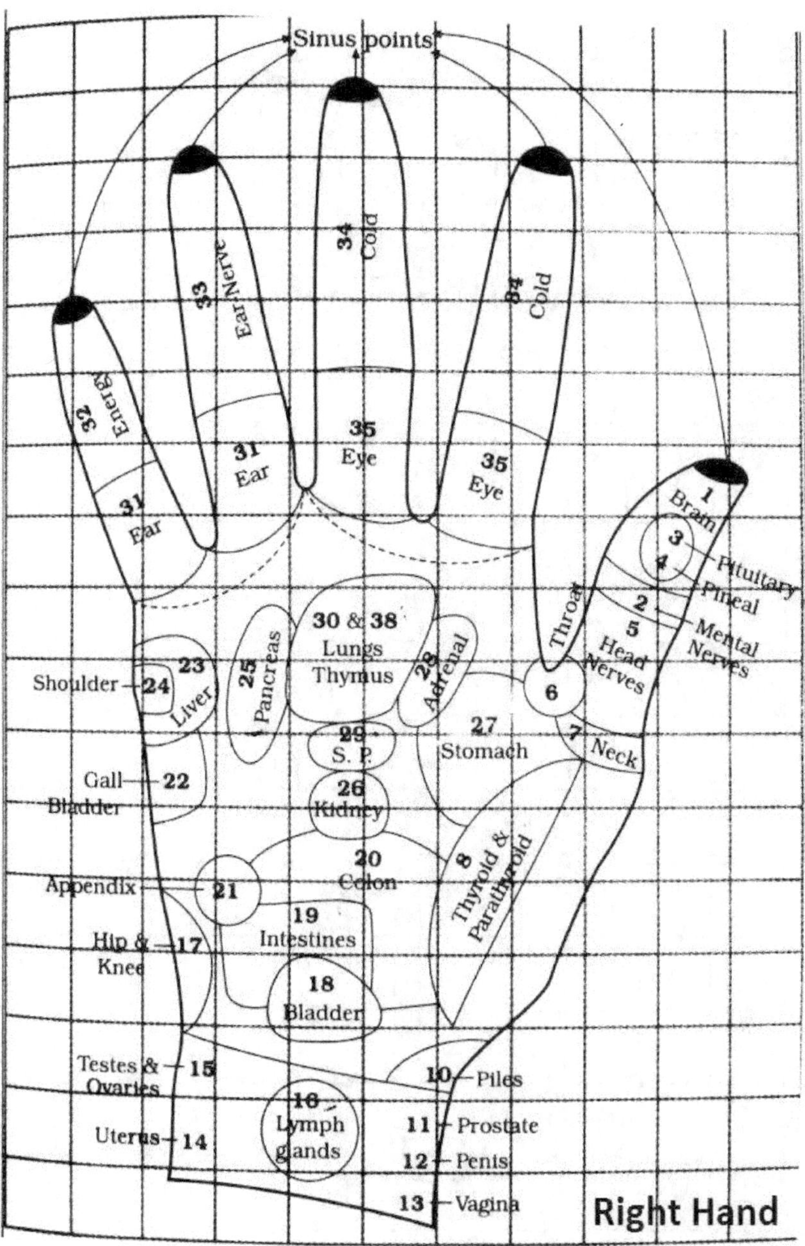

Right Foot

Sinus points
1 — Brain
3 — Pituitary
4 — Pineal
2 — Mental nerves
5 — Head nerves
Throat
34
34
Cold
Cold
Cold
33
Ear nerve
35
Eye
6
7 Neck
32
31
Energy
Ear
8
Thyroid & Parathyroid
30 & 38
Lungs & Thymus
23
29 — Solar Plexus
Shoulder — 24 Liver
Gall bladder
22
Pancreas — 25
27 28 9 — Spine
Stomach — Adrenal
Kidney
26
Colon 20
19
Intestines
16 — Lower lumbar
Appendix — 21
18
Bladder
Hip & Knee
17
10 Piles

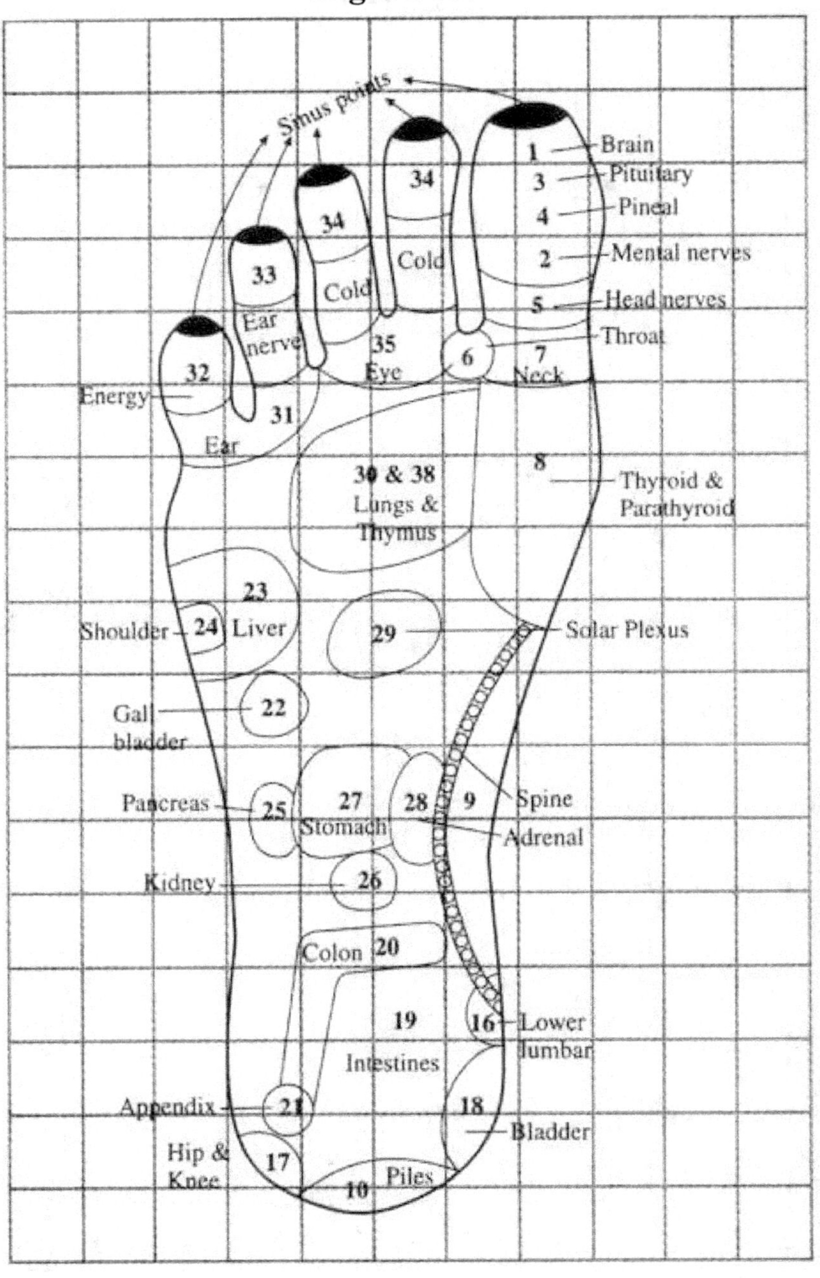

Left Foot

Sirus points
Brain 1
Pituitary 3
Pineal 4
Mental nerves 2
Head nerves 5
Throat 6
7 Neck
34 Cold
34 Cold
35 Eye
33 Ear nerve
32
31 Ear
Energy
Thyroid & Parathyroid 8
30 & 38 Lungs & Thymus
36 Heart
24 Shoulder
Solar Plexus
29
Spleen
37
28
27 Stomach
Adrenal
25 Pancreas
Spine 9
26 Kidney
20 Colon
Lower lumbar 16
19
Intestines
Bladder 18
17 Hip & Knee
Piles 10

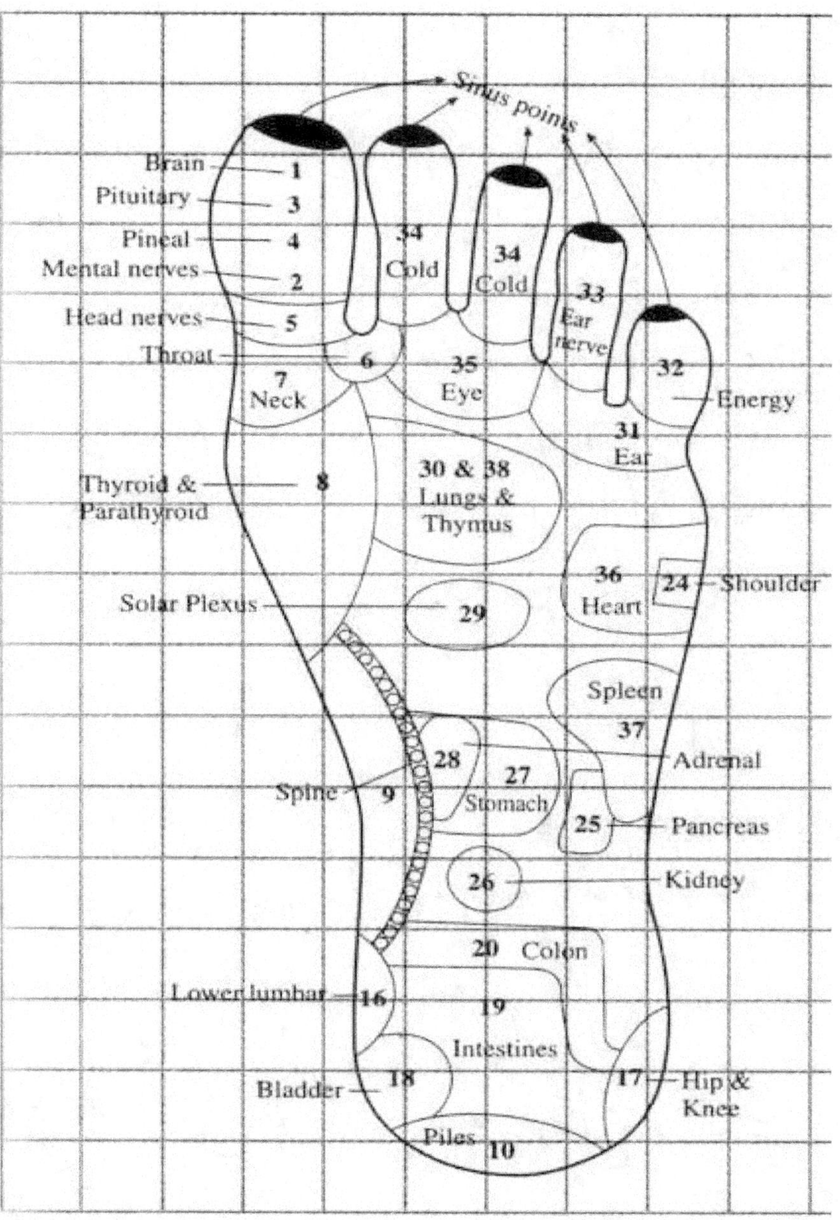

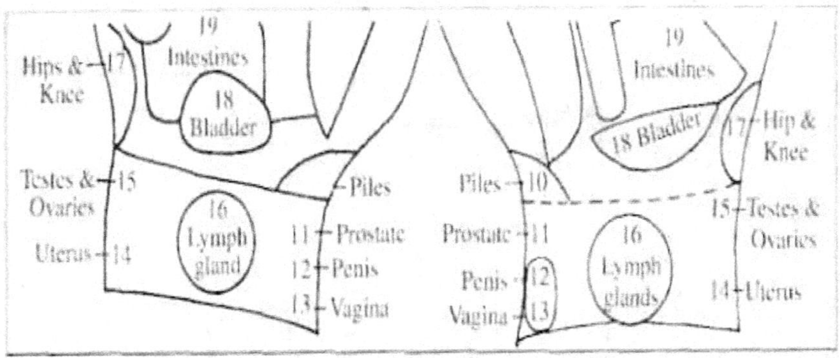

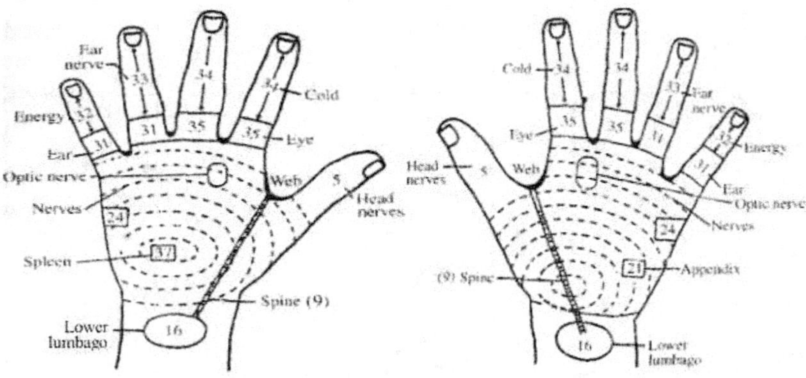

**Fig. 18 (a): Back
Side of Left Hand**

**Fig. 18 (b): Back
Side of Right Hand**

Fig. 19 (a): Inside of Foot

Fig. 19 (b): Outside of Foot

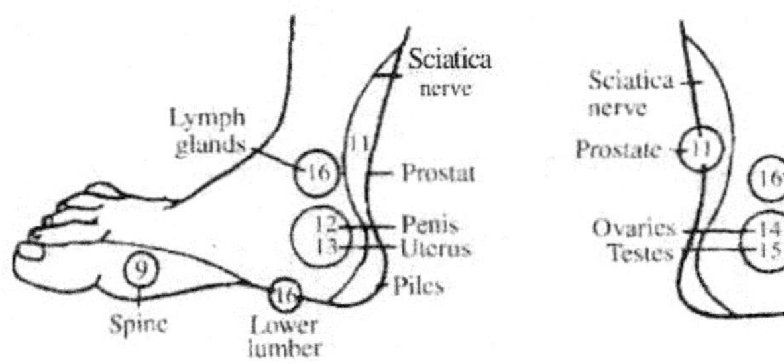

Urinary System

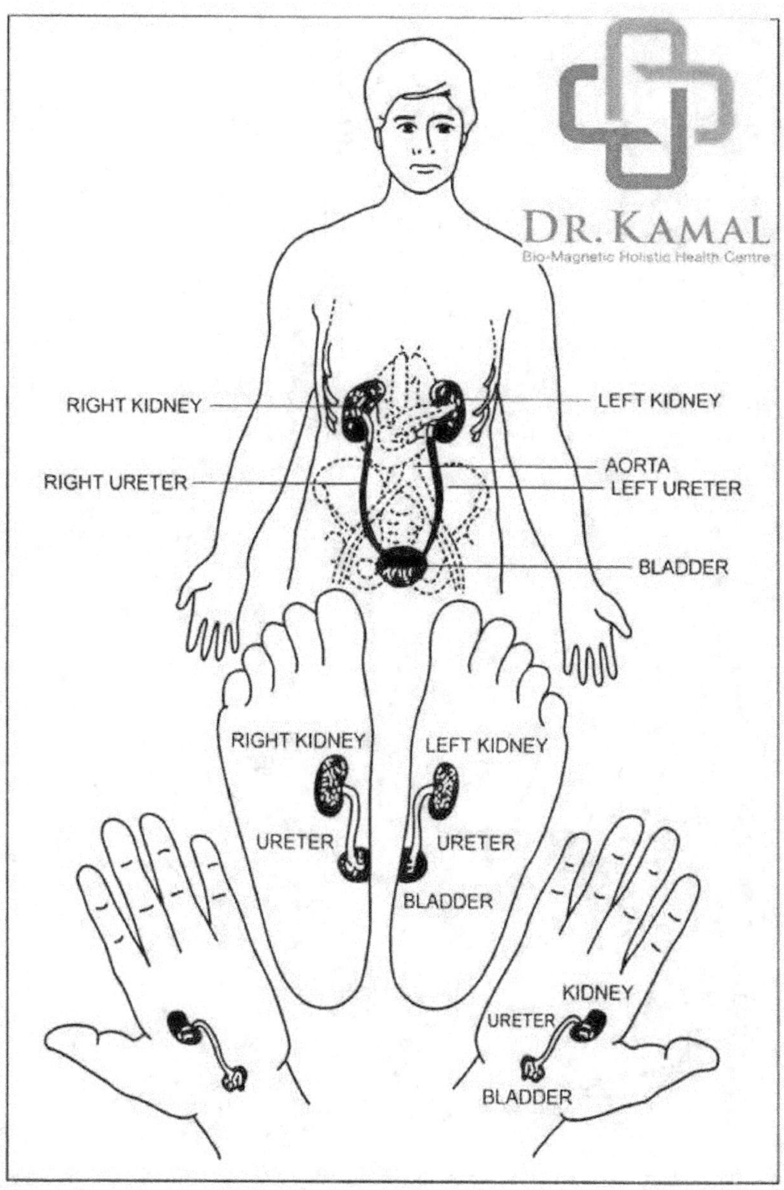

Nervous System, Eye, Ear and Skeletal System

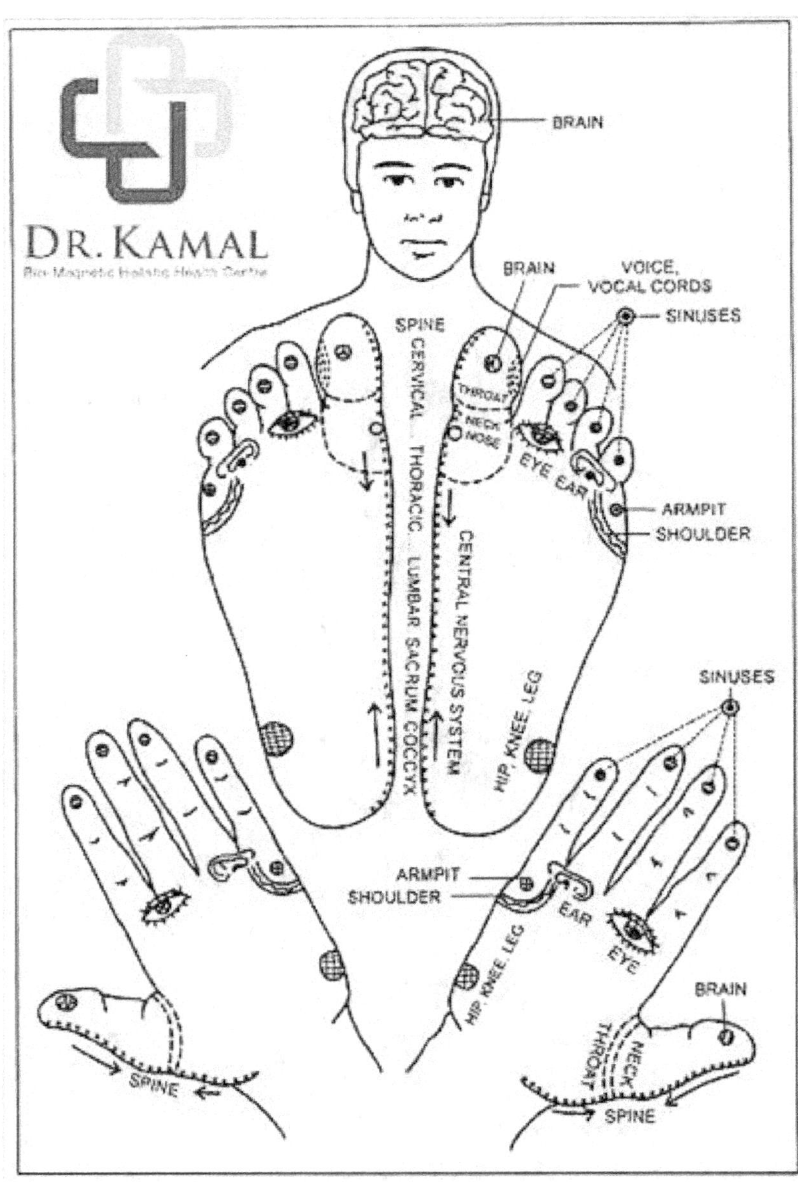

Reproductive System

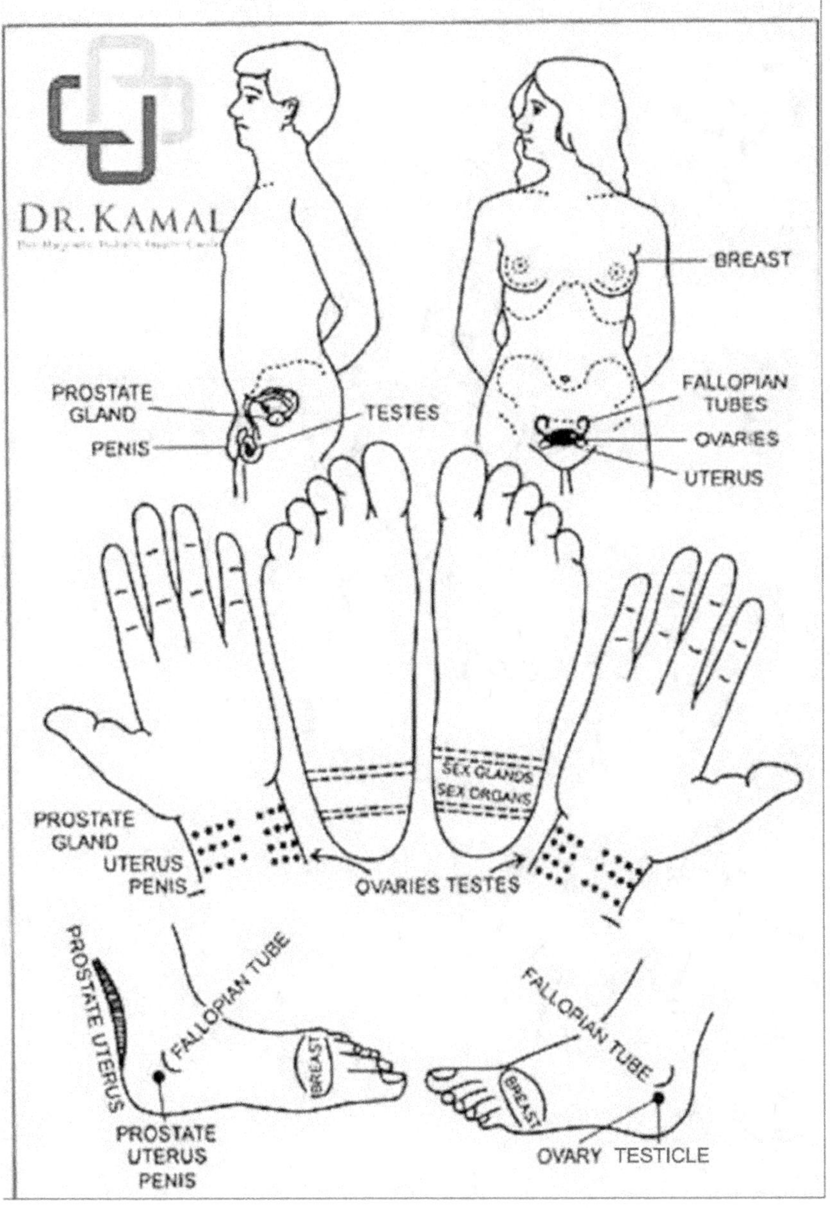

Respiratory System

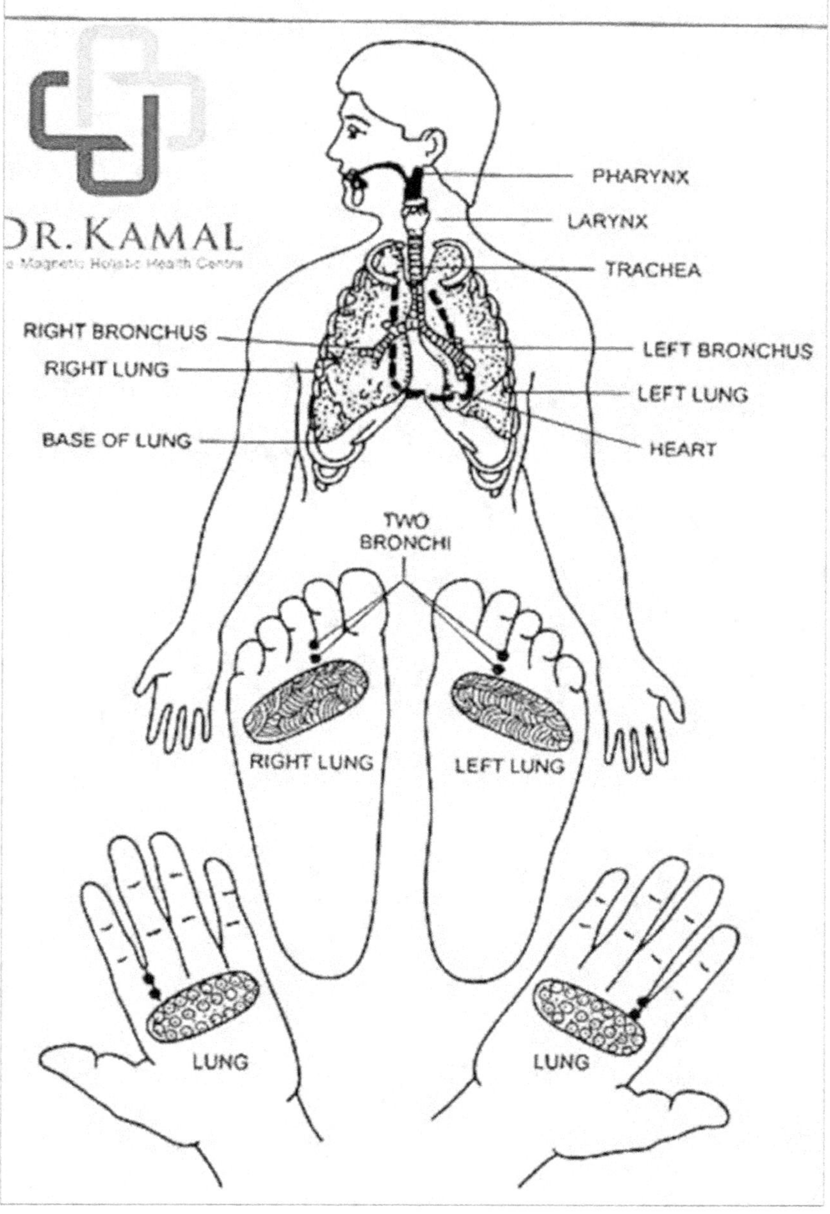

Functions and Effects of the Malfunctioning of Endocrine Glands

Name of the Gland	Effects of Malfunctioning
1. **Thymus Gland (No. 38):** - Protects the child up to the age of 15 years.	Child gets sick. In case the gland becomes active later on it brings dullness.
2. **Pineal Gland (No. 4):** -Controls sex system and water of the body. It's a Primitive Eye.	Premature sex development, increase in water content, high blood pressure.
3. **Pituitary Gland (No. 3):** - It's the king of glands and controls the other glands. Governs the brain and development of the body.	Body becomes dwarfish or bulging. Produces mental retardation. Child becomes bully, or a liar and disobedient.
4. **Thyroid/Parathyroid (No. 8):** - Para Thyroid gland controls digestion of calcium in the body, also controls the development of the body.	Underworking leads to rickets, convulsion, and teeth problems, twisting of muscles, fatness and dullness. Overworking leads in over growth, bulging of the eyes. Adam's apple, stone in the kidney, etc.
5. **Adrenal Gland (No. 28):** - Controls production of biles, liver and also the flow of blood, blood pressure it also molds character	Underworking leads to dullness, timidness, less energy, less oxygenation. Overworking leads to high B.P., migraine, headache, less bile leads to acidity, vomiting and severe headache.
6. **Pancreas (Point No. 25):** - Controls digestion of sugar in the body and digestive juices.	Underworking leads to diabetes and overworking leads to low B.P., dizziness and even to alcoholism through Hypoglycemia (Shortage of Sugar in the body)

7. Ovaries, Testes & Sex Glands (No. 14- 15): - Controls digestion of phosphorus and heat of the body, attractiveness and productive side of the body.	Reproductive organs are damaged, problem of less or more menses, self-abuse, loss of heat leading to development of fat. Un- attractiveness of the body, less/more sex desire.
8. Lymph Gland (No. 16): - Stops formation of pus and prevents germs.	Disease called Lymphocytosis leads to increase in blood sugar

Endocrine System

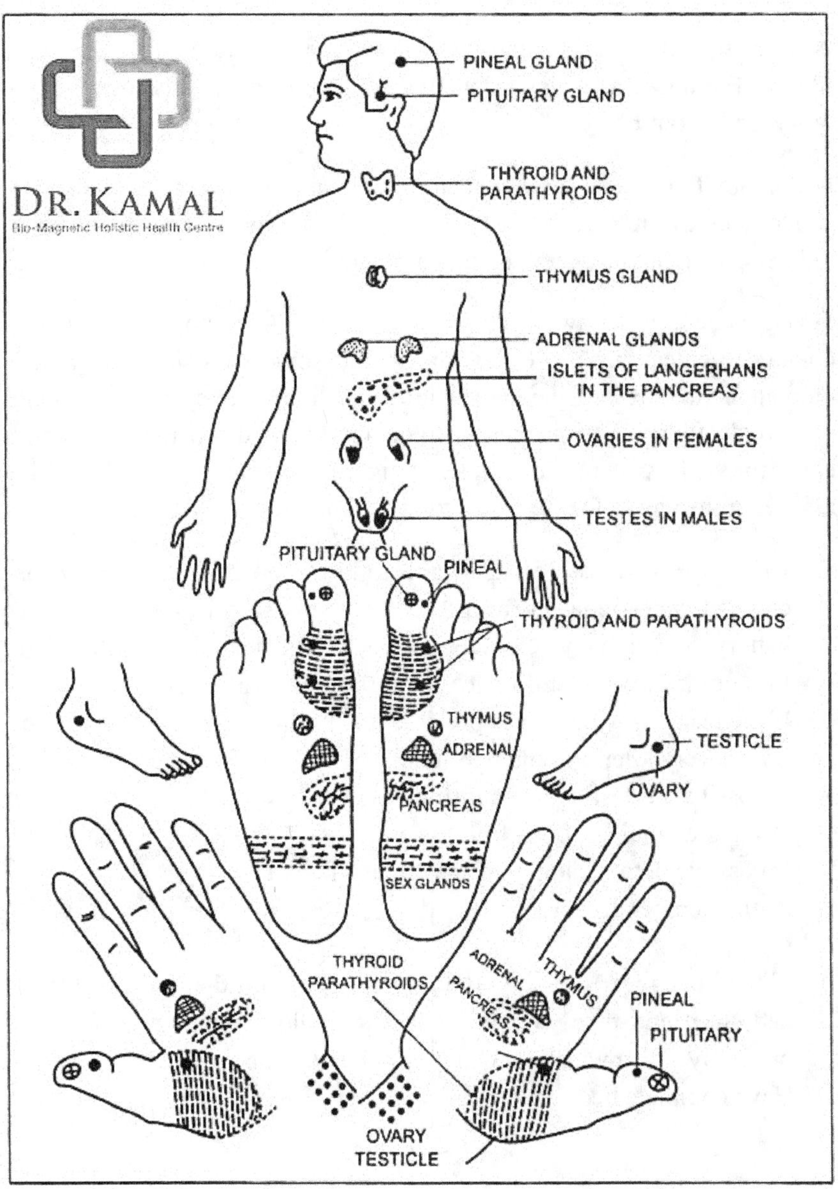

HOW TO FIND OUT ABOUT THE TYPE OF FEVER

A fever is a temporary increase in your body temperature, often due to an illness. Having a fever is a sign that something out of the ordinary is going on in your body.

For an adult, a fever may be uncomfortable, but usually isn't a cause for concern unless it reaches 103 F (39.4 C) or higher. For infants and toddlers, a slightly elevated temperature may indicate a serious infection.

Fevers generally go away within a few days. A number of over-the-counter medications lower a fever, but sometimes it's better left untreated. Fever is a very good friend, seems to play a key role in helping your body fight off a number of infections, burn down the toxins and clean the body system. So instead of fighting against him, it should be assisted in its work. The best way to assist it is to;

1. Drink 3 to 4 glasses of lukewarm to hot – Gold/Silver/Copper/Iron charged water reduced from 8 to 6 glasses. This will empower the battery of the body. Gold is a very efficient antibiotic; therefore further medicine of antibiotic will not be necessary.
2. If the charged water is not possible, then drink only one glass of hot water every after one and half hour.
3. If possible do fasting, refrain from foods.
4. Drink green juices, fresh fruit juices.
5. If possible detox colon with any Nature T infusion.
6. If the temperature rises 102 degree keep ice packs on head & stomach.
7. If the high fever crossing 103 degree; cover up the body with wet bed sheet and then woolen blanket and allow perspiration to flow profusely. Then wipe it out and keep the body dry.
8. Have complete bed rest.

In order to have further proper treatment, it is necessary to find out about the type of fever. So press different points on Palm/Soles if there is pain on the reflex points.

Point No.	It Denotes/Symptoms
6	Throat – It could be tonsillitis.
30	**Congestion** – could be bronchitis
37	**Malaria** – It's obvious as the patient gets fever after a short bout of shivering, fever up shoots and comes on alternative days. There is sweating and the loss of healthy red blood cells results in anemia.
19	**Typhoid** – It could be typhoid, causing general weakness, high fever, chills, sweating, inflammation of spleen and bones.
23	**Jaundice** – Liver is badly damaged
16	**Infection** – There is some infection in the body.
16 + 26	**Infection in Kidney**
16 + 37	**Advanced Infection in the Blood** – Could be due to degeneration **(Cancer)** in the blood or advanced case of **AIDS**
16 + 1 to 5	**Meningitis** – Causing an intense headache, fever, loss of appetite, convulsions, vomiting and delirium.
16 + 6	**Fever due to Cancer in mouth** – Could be in gums, teeth, cheeks or throat.
16 + 11 to 15	**Due to infection – Cancerous effects** (males), and in Uterus, Vagina (females).
16 + 30	**T.B., Pneumonia** – There is fever, feeling of uneasiness, headache etc., together with cough and chest pain.

In any of these fevers, ask the patient not to worry, but take proper treatment as mentioned in the book.

ਨਵਕਿਰਨ ਚੁੰਬਕੀ ਕਲੀਨਿਕ

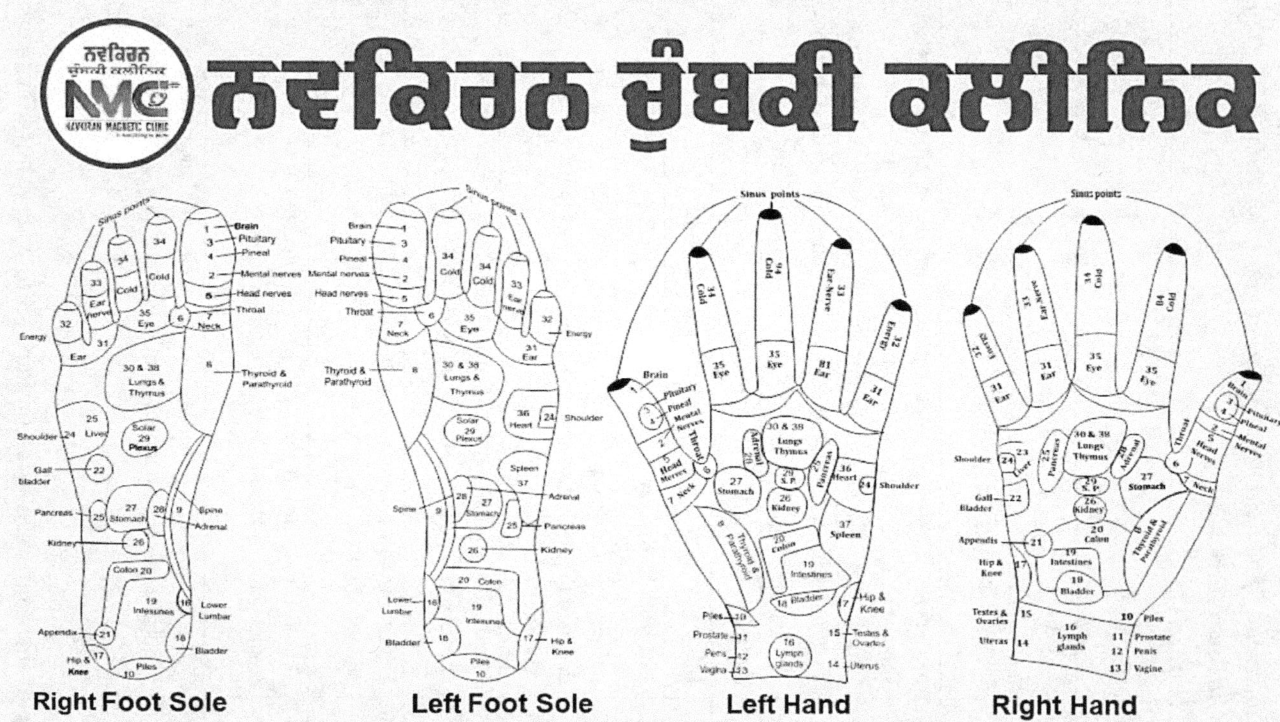

COMMON DISEASES

In Neuro Acupressure therapy it is an accepted fact that our body is so wonderful, it reveals all its problems. There is no need to study the symptoms or names of diseases. Even it is not necessary to go long details about the past history, because any problem even though it may be just in the beginning stage, the corresponding/reflex points on the palms/soles become tender and so when you press there, can feel the pain/reflection.

It is easy to find out which organ has been damaged. In the acupressure Pictures of hands and feet there are 39 points, which are related to different working organs. In case of problem of Liver, Point No. 23 has to be pressed. While in case of trouble in the right eye, Point No. 35 on right palm has to be pressed. For easy diagnosis this process has to be reversed. That is for example, for any eye problem like watering, redness or pain will be diagnosed when you press on Point No. 35 and observe hurting on it. So whether the patient tell you about his eye problem or not while checking his/her palms, if you observe any hurting, even a flicker in the eyes, when you press on Point No. 35 of right palm- you can tell the patient that he/she has a problem in the right eye. At the same time, also press Point No. 35 on left palm and if there is hurting or flickering such problem also exists in the left eye. To go further also press Point No. 39 Optic Nerve on the back of both hands, if there is hurting it denotes that the patient has a problem in retina of his/her eyes. Now you are aware that the optic nerve is controlled by the Pituitary Gland. So to get confirmation about the damage to the retina, you are supposed to press on Point No. 3 on both the thumbs, and surprisingly you will observe hurting on Point No. 3. Thus you are able to diagnose not only the common eye problem of the patient but even any other such serious problem.

When you locate such serious problem, go deeper to find out the root cause.

Thus diagnosis of all types of common ailments is very easy – when there is a hurting pain, when you press on……

Point No.	It Denotes
1-2-5	**Headache:** Cold in head
3-4	**High Blood Pressure:** High BP/ malfunctioning of Pineal, Pituitary (refer to the previous chapters and understand their effects of less or Overworking.)
1-2-3-4-5 & 16	**Brain:** In such a case there will be hurting pain on Point No. 8 – 28 and points of other endocrine glands.
6	**Throat**
6 + 16	**Serious Problem in Throat-** It may be cancerous effect.
7	**Pain behind the Neck –** Spondylitis
8	**Barometer of the body -** It indicates something wrong somewhere in the body.
More Pain on 8	**Deficiency of Calcium –** In the case of overworking, it creates calcification leading to stones.
Pain on 8 + 26	**Kidney Stones.**
8 + 16	**Hypothyroidism -** Subnormal activity of Thyroid gland. Weight gain, undue sensitivity to cold, slowing of the pulse, coarsening of the skin, mental and physical slowing.

8 + 11	**Cause for Obesity** – A condition in which excess fat has accumulated in the body, resulting low vitality.
9	**Spondylitis** – Stiff neck **Lower Back** – Lower Lumbar
Could also be damage to sciatic Nerve, So confirm it by pressing on the point of Sciatic Nerve on legs	**Lower Lumbar – Knee Pain, Numbness and weakness in legs from waist towards toes. Damages to sciatic nerve leading to sensation, muscle weakness – slipped disc.**

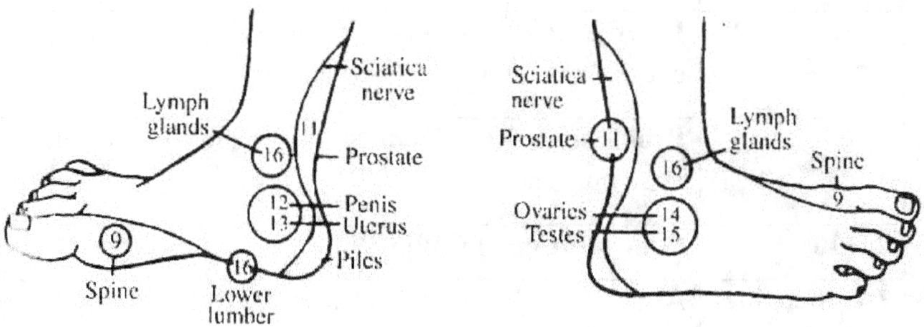

9 + 37 + 16	**Degeneration of Bones**
9 + 11 to 15	**Backache due to Sex Problems** – (Both males and females)
10	**Piles** – (in this case check solar plexus and correct it.
11	**Prostate** – Frequent urination during the day and or night.
11 to 15	**Sex Problems** – (In both males and females) (Pimples, Less or More Menses, Painful Menses, Irregular Menses, Timidity, Loss of Libido, Less Virility (Check the Nails)

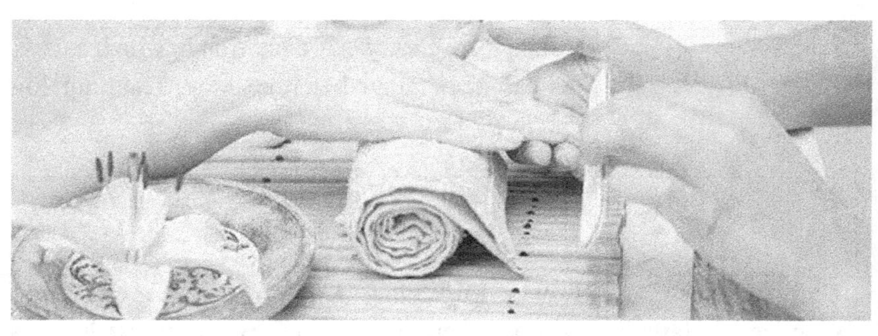

11 to 15 + 16	**Degeneration of Prostate or V.D. (in males)** **Degeneration of Uterus (in females)**
17	**Pain in Hips and Knees**
18	**Problem in Bladder** – Trouble in passing urine or excess storage of urine
19	**Problem in Intestine**
19+22+23+28	**Ulcer – Acidity – Gas Trouble** – If pain persists, check the mouth as there could be ulcer.
20	**Problem about Colon** – The main part of the large intestine
20+16	**Degeneration of Colon**
21(inner side of Palm)	**Appendix** – It also indicates early development of this problem.
21 (Back of Palm)	**Allergy**
21+8	**Allergy plus deficiency of Calcium**
22 – 23	**Problem in Gallbladder plus Liver** –an early indication of **Jaundice.**
More pain on 22-23	**Jaundice** – indication of **Crystallization** of biles in gallbladder (**Considered to be Stone in Gallbladder**)
23+16	**Degeneration of Liver**

Point	Condition
24	**Stiffness in Shoulder**
9+24	**Frozen Shoulder**
25	**Malfunctioning of Pancreas** – Overworking leads to migraine, desire to eat-drink sweets and later on to alcoholism.
25+28	**Under working of Pancreas**
25+28+16	**Diabetes**
26	**All problems related to Kidneys**
26+25	**Skin problem**
26+4	**Retention of fluid**
26+8	**Stone in Kidney**
27	**Stomach** – Loss of appetite, digestion problem, gas trouble.
28	**Problem related to Adrenal Gland** – Excess heat in the body. Depression, fear of more pain, severe depression indicates desire to commit suicide (suicidal tendency), less circulation of blood and so less oxygenation.
29	**Solar Plexus** – If shifted upward leads to Constipation, Hiatus Hernia- Piles – Fistula; if shifted downwards, leads to Loose Motion. Colitis- inflammation of colon, leading to diarrhea and lower abdominal pain.
30	**Lung Problem**
30+6	**Bronchitis** – Even fever due to it.
30+16+8	**T.B.**
31	**Ear Problem** – Less hearing etc.
31+28	**Cold around Ears** – Due to excess heat.
31+Point for worms+16	**Ear infection due to worms**
31+16+33	**Frequent Noise in the Ears – Even Vertigo**

32	Less Energy – Low Vitality.
34+27	Common Cold affecting the nose, throat and bronchial tubes.
34+28	Cold due to excess heat
34+8+6	Tonsils
35	Problems of redness of eyes, watering of eyes.
35+ (Optic Nerve) +3 & 4 + Pain in Eyes	Beginning of damage to retina. Advanced stage of damage to retina, could be glaucoma, a condition in which the pressure within the eyeball causes dimness and ultimately loss of Vision.

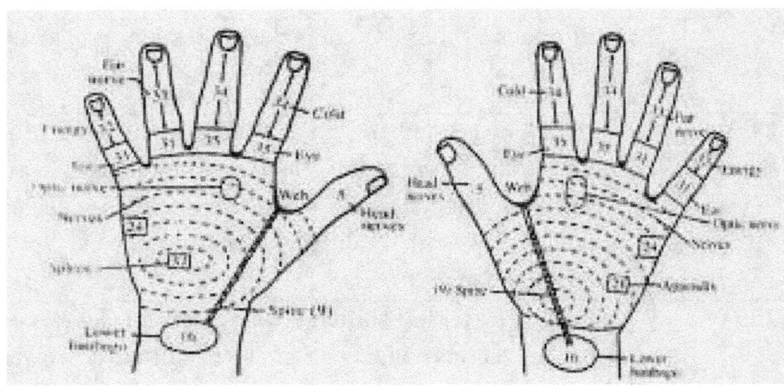

(Optic Nerve Points)

36	Heart – Problems related to Heart.
36+28	Poor Circulation of Blood
36+8	Could be Heart Attack
36+8+ breathlessness	Varicose Veins, Blockage in arteries.
37	Problem of Spleen – anemia, (Check the point of worms)

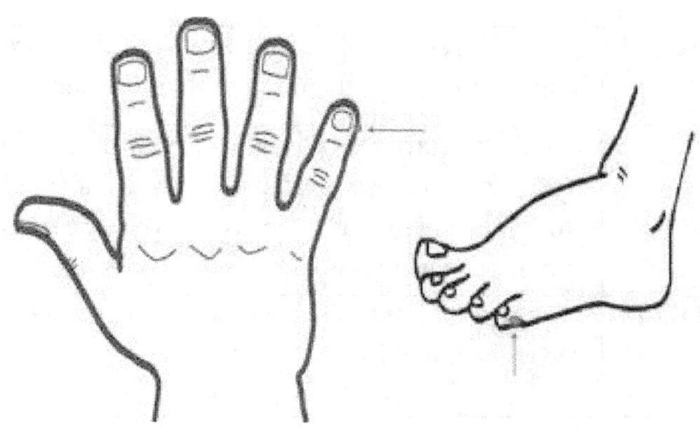

Easy Technique to check for Intestinal Worms

37+16 (wrist side)	Degeneration of Blood.
37+16 (Back of Palm) +9	Degeneration of blood and bones

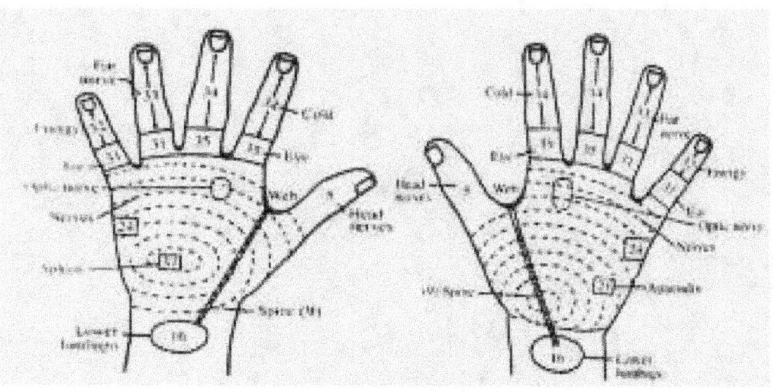

37	**Patient looking healthy could be HIV affected-** therefore call for partner and children below 15 and if such pain found in partner it could be **HIV**
37+11 to 15	**HIV due to sex abuse, multiple sex partners and unnatural sex,** could be VD or any other diseases transmitted by sexual intercourse, **(In Case of VD** There may be burning sensation while urinating.

37+22+23+28	**In Children Thalassemia** – Call the parents and siblings and check them too to find out the root cause.
38	**Problem related to Thymus** – In the case of children - weakened defense system. In case of adult; Over working of Thymus – leads to Myasthenia gravis, a condition causing loss of muscle power.
In the middle of right arm	**Weakened Valve of Energy Flow** – leading to decaying and old age.

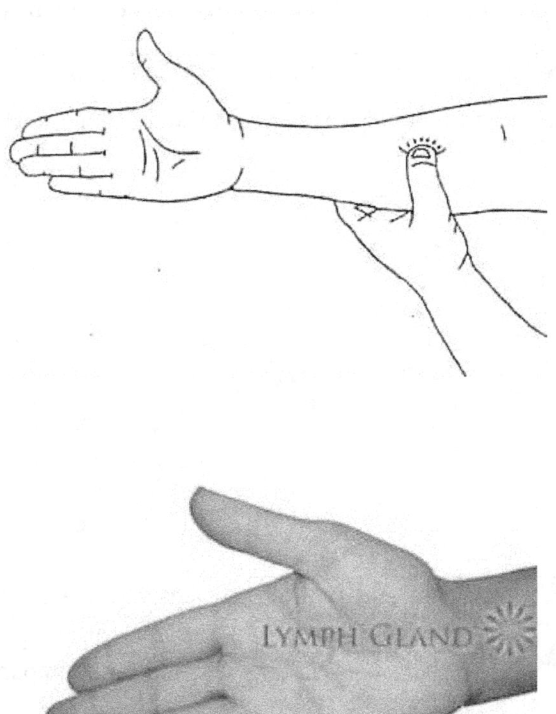

16 (Front Side) as shown in the picture below	Diabetes – Infection – Boils etc.
16 + 25	**Diabetes** – over 2% - 200 in blood Plus sugar in urine leading to thirst, loss of weight and excessive production of urine.
16 + 31	**Infection of Ears.**
16 + 26	**Infection of Kidney**
16 + 11 to 15	**Infection of the sex organs – prostate, penis or uterus leading to degeneration + V.D.**
16 + 11 to 15 + on back of right palm (middle)	**Degeneration of Prostate (in males).** **Degeneration of Uterus (in females).** **Degeneration of Uterus + right breast**
16 + 11 to 15 + on back of left palm middle	**Degeneration of Uterus + left breast.**

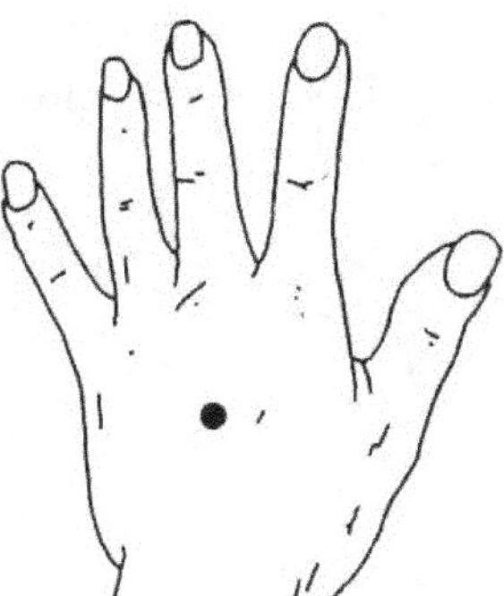

Back of Left Palm

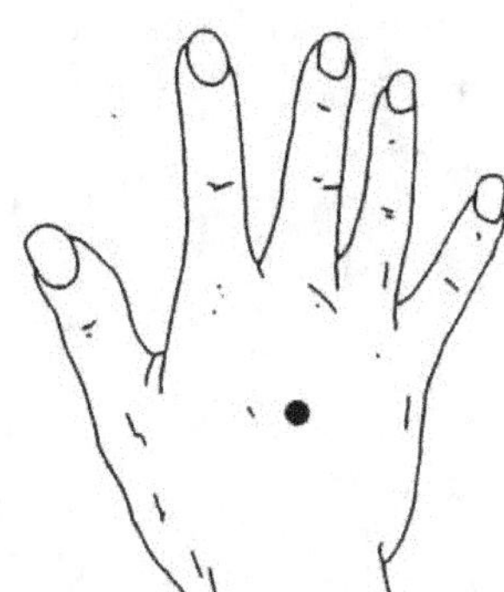

Back of Right Palm

16 + 6	Degeneration of Teeth, Tongue and Throat
16 + point between 6 & 27	Degeneration of windpipe (causing difficulty in swallowing)
16 + 27	Degeneration of Stomach
16 + 19	Degeneration of Small Intestine
16 + 20	Degeneration of Large Intestine
16 + 22 + 23	Degeneration of Gall Bladder & Liver
16 + 30	Degeneration of Lungs (T.B.)
16 + 1 to 5	Destruction of healthy Brain cells (Could be Tumor of brain)
16 + 37	Degeneration of Blood
16 + 37 + 9	Degeneration of Blood + Bones

(In the case of pain of Point No. 37, first checkup if there are any boils, pus formation in cuts/ear infection etc.)

If not, get the medical checkup done of urine and blood sugar. If no sugar found in urine or blood means no diabetes, then it's a clear indication about degeneration. But the Practitioner/Patient needs not to worry. Assure the patient that all types of degenerations are curable.

In the same way even in case of V.D. and HIV or Thalassemia, assure the patient that if proper treatment is taken for 60-75 days it helps speedy recovery and cure.

ACIDITY – GASTRIC TROUBLE

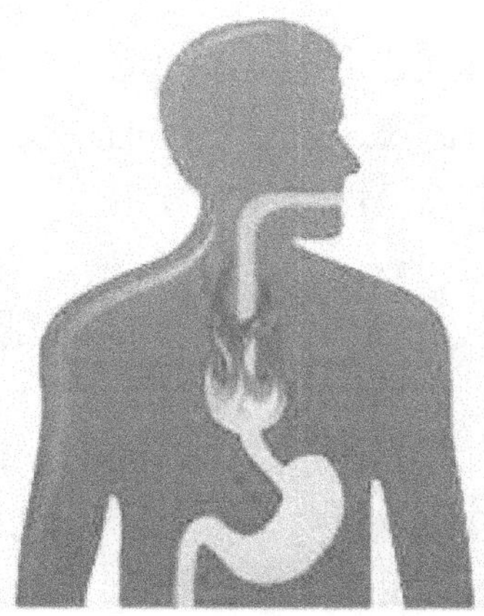

The food we eat goes into our stomach through the esophagus. The gastric glands in your stomach create acid, which is necessary to digest the food. When the gastric glands create more acid than needed for the digestion process, you can feel a burning sensation below the breastbone. This condition is commonly known as acidity.

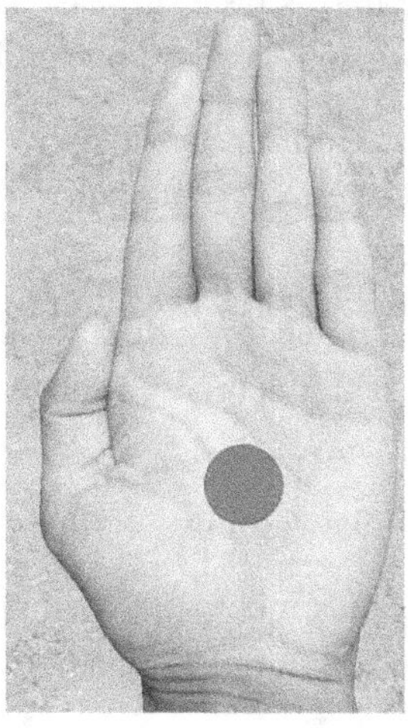

Use your left hand in this acupressure. The green mark on the hand in the picture is the acupressure point for the Acidity. Also rub from bottom to up.

Causes of acidity: -

Acidity is caused due to excess production of acid in the stomach by the gastric glands. Factors that cause acidity include:

- Unhealthy eating habits
- Skipping meals or eating at irregular times
- Eating just before sleeping
- Overeating
- Consumption of spicy food
- High intake of table salt
- Diet low in dietary fiber

Home remedies for acidity: -

- Coconut water: This tasty treat is known to soothe your stomach and the digestive system. Take at least two glasses a day.
- Watermelon juice: It is great to counter acidity. You can take a glass of watermelon juice with breakfast.
- Fresh lime juice that is taken at least an hour before lunch helps to reduce the uneasiness caused by acidity.
- A glass of buttermilk after a spicy meal helps reduce the uneasiness as buttermilk contains lactic acid that normalises acidity in the stomach
- You can either munch on a few basil leaves, or boil them in water and drink it frequently to reduce acid reflux. You can also do this with mint leaves.
- Drink a glass of lukewarm water after every meal
- Include banana, cucumber and yoghurt in your diet. They are known to give instant relief from acidity.
- Surprisingly, sucking on a piece of clove when you have acidity helps to reduce the symptoms.

+ Ginger aids in digestion. Use ginger in your cooking or boil it in a glass of water, reduce to half glass and consume the water.

+ Cumin is a great remedy for acidity. Munch on some cumin or boil a teaspoon of cumin in a glass of water. Boil until the water is reduced to half. Drink it on an empty stomach.

+ Try chewing gum! As unbelievable as it may sound, chewing gum generates saliva that helps to move the food through the esophagus.

+ Take a tablespoon of apple cider vinegar with a glass of water every morning on an empty stomach.

+ Drink at least two liters of water every day.

BREATHING DIFFICULTIES

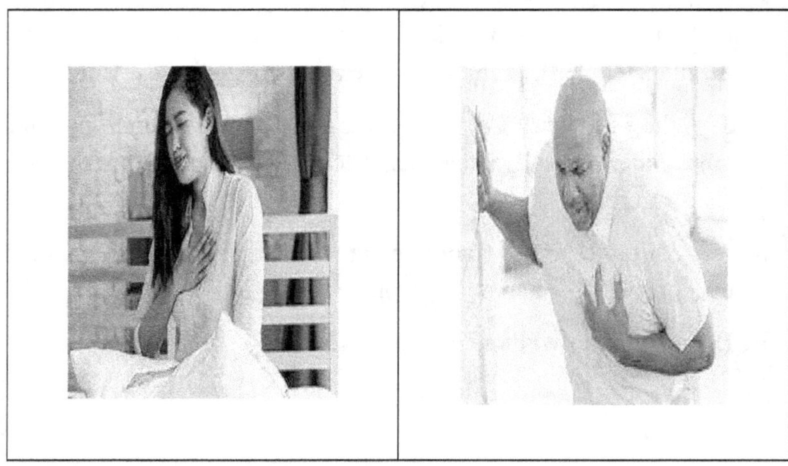

Experiencing breathing difficulty describes discomfort when breathing and feeling as if you can't draw a complete breath. This can develop gradually or come on suddenly. Mild breathing problems, such as fatigue after an aerobics class, don't fall into this category.

Breathing difficulties can be caused by many different conditions. They can also develop as a result of stress and anxiety. It's important to note that frequent episodes of shortness of breath or sudden, intense breathing difficulty may be signs of a serious health issue that needs medical attention. You should discuss any breathing concerns with your doctor.

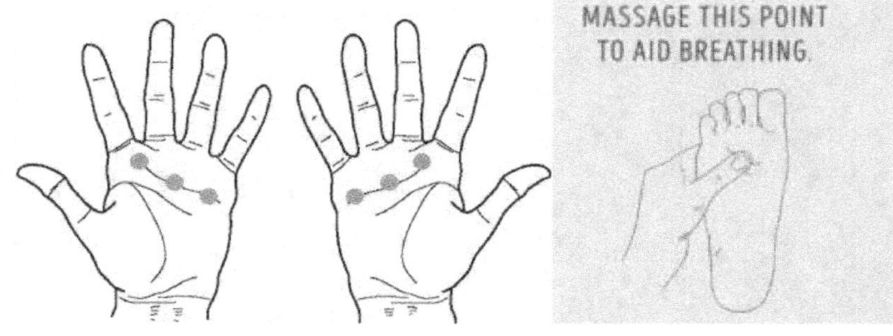

Apply Pressure on these Points

Home Remedies:

- When you begin to feel short of breath, stop what you are doing and rest until your breathing returns to normal.

- Instead of focusing on your breathing, try to distract your mind. This helps your subconscious mind take control of your breathing again.

- Take short breaks at regular intervals while doing strenuous activities to avoid shortness of breath.

- Avoid exposure to toxic chemicals at home or work. Eat a diet full of fruits and vegetables.

- Drink plenty of water to keep your body hydrated and thin out the mucus, making it easier to expel.

- Do not take any supplement or medicine without consulting your doctor.

- People with asthma may use an inhaler before exercising.

- Use a humidifier, especially in winter, as dry air thickens mucus and can make breathing difficult.

COUGH AND COLD

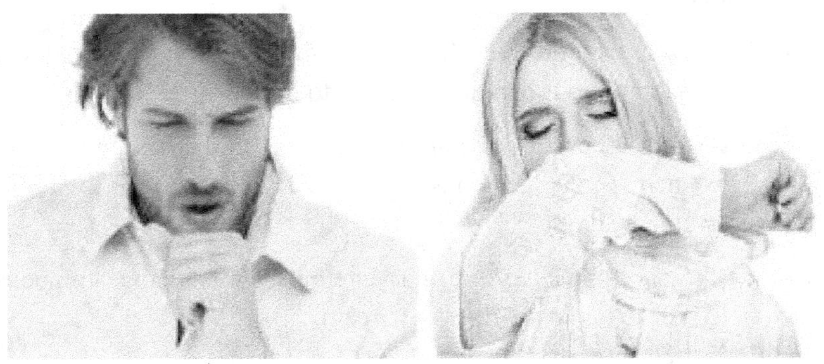

Coughs and colds are common diseases in children caused by germs or viruses. Colds are fast spreading viral diseases of the soft lining of the nose called the mucosa. These normally ease up at their own, and antibiotic medicines are usually of no use. It is said that cough and cold gets cured at its own in 4-10 days. However, if the symptoms still persist than it can be something else. Cold is also seasonal, it is most common during winter season and affects children mostly because they have a lower immunity.

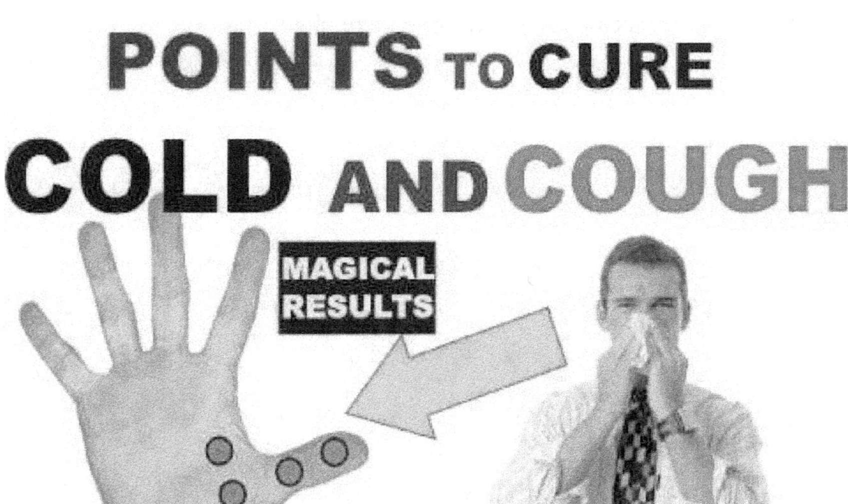

Home Remedies: -

- Turmeric Milk
- Giloy Juice
- Honey + Mulethi + Cinnamon
- Black Pepper
- Pomegranate Juice for Kids
- Spiced Tea

DIABETES

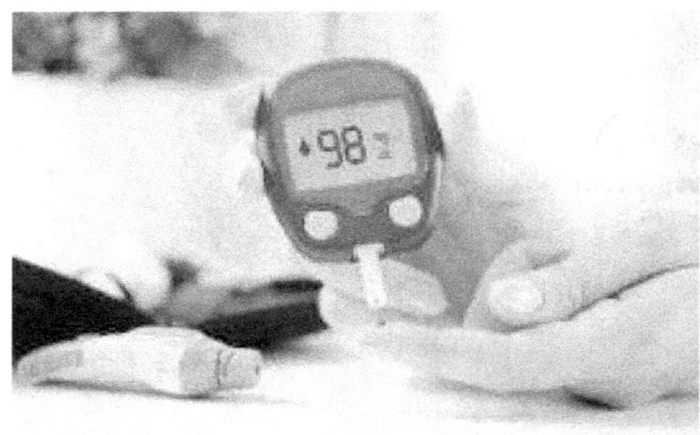

Diabetes is a disease in which the body's ability to produce or respond to the hormone insulin is impaired, resulting in abnormal metabolism of carbohydrates and elevated levels of glucose in the blood and urine.

Wrist-Hand Pressure Point The spot found quickly and lies on the side of the little finger near the wrist. By massaging the point, it helps relieve stress from your heart and controls diabetes automatically.

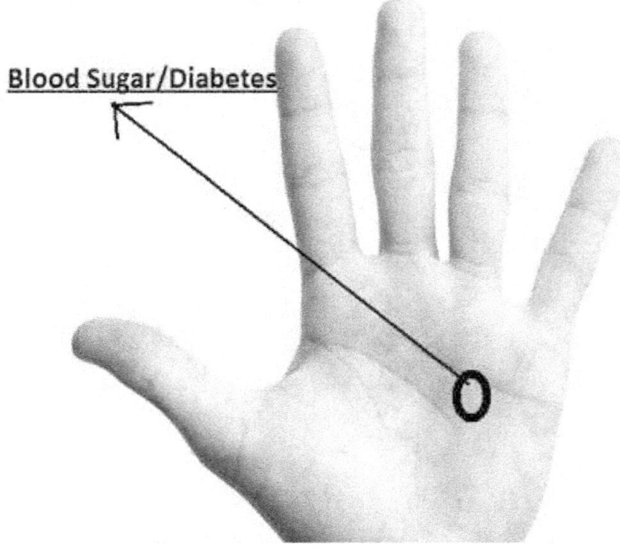

- **BITTER GOURD OR KARELA:** Rich in plant insulin-polypeptide-P, bitter gourd or karela have the ability to reduce the hyperglycemia (increase in sugar levels). Bitter gourd also contains two very essential compounds called charatin and momordicin, which are the key compounds in lowering one's blood sugar levels.
  - Consume karela once a week withers as a sabzi or in a curry.
  - Slice the bitter gourd and scrape away the flesh to remove the seeds. Add the sliced vegetable to a blender and run till it becomes juice. Drink one small glass of this juice on empty stomach every morning.
- **FENUGREEK:** Fenugreek is a commonly used herb in Indian kitchen with great many benefits. It is helps to control diabetes, improve glucose tolerance, lower blood sugar levels and stimulate the secretion of glucose- dependent insulin.
  - Soak 2 tbsp. of fenugreek seeds in water overnight and drink that water along with the seeds in the morning in an empty stomach daily to bring down your glucose level.
  - Consume fenugreek seed powder with hot or cold water or milk daily.
- **MANGO LEAVES:** Fresh mango leaves are an effective home remedy to manage and treat diabetes.
  - Wash and sun-dry tender mango leaves and grind to powder. Consume this powder with water at morning and night daily.
  - Boil some fresh mango leaves in a glass of water and leave it to cool overnight. Drink the water in the morning on empty stomach.
- **INDIAN GOOSEBERRY OR AMLA:** Indian gooseberry or amla is one of the richest sources of vitamin C and helps your pancreas to produce optimum so that your blood glucose levels remain balanced.

> Discard the seeds and grind 2-3 amla into fine paste and squeeze out its juice. Mix this juice (approximately 2 tbsp.) in cup of water and drink it every morning n empty stomach.
> Mix a cup of bitter gourd juice and 1 tbsp. of amla juice and drink it daily.
> Consume raw amla every day

✦ DRUMSTICK OR MORINGA LEAVES; The drumstick or moringa oleifera leaves are best known for its ability to Drumstick or Moringa oleifera leaves are best known for its ability to maintain blood sugar levels and boost one's energy. The moringa leaves contain nutrients which increases the insulin secretion in the body. The leaves are also rich in antioxidants and have anti-inflammatory properties.

Include 50 grams of fresh moringa leaves to a meal. It will not only add a flavor but also reduce the rise in blood sugar by 21%. Either toss them like a salad or steam them like spinach.

✦ SUNLIGHT: In recent years, researchers have linked low Vitamin D levels to insulin resistance and diabetes. Studies found that Vitamin D plays a vital role in the production on insulin in the body. The lower your levels of vitamin D, the more prone you are to develop type 2 diabetes.

> Expose yourself to 30 minutes of daily sun to avoid Vitamin D deficiency.
> Include Vitamin D rich foods in your daily diet such as orange juice, soy milk, cheese, yogurt and cereals.

✦ WATER: For people with diabetes, the risk of dehydration is greater. To get rid of the glucose, the kidneys will try to pass it out in the urine, but that takes water. So the higher your blood glucose, the more fluids you should drink, which is why thirst is one of the main symptoms of diabetes.

> Consume 2.5 liters of water a day.

EYES PROBLEMS

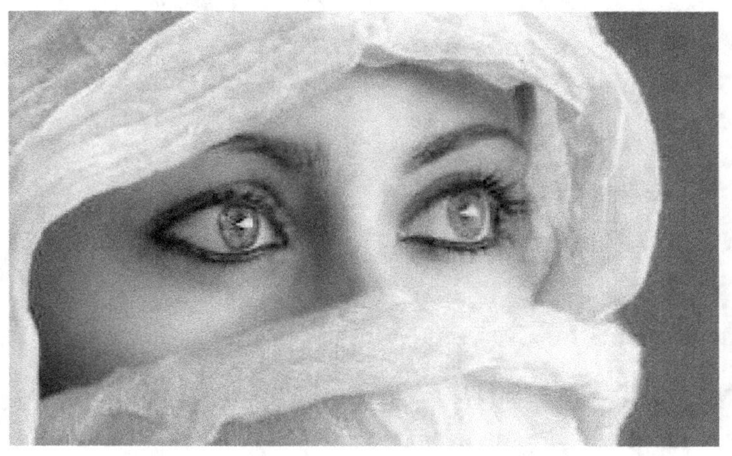

Your eyes are the parts of your body with which you see. Following are the diseases of the eyes;

- ➢ Myopia – Short Sight.
- ➢ Hypermetropia- Long Sight
- ➢ Presbyopia- Old age Sight
- ➢ Glaucoma
- ➢ Cataract
- ➢ Night Blindness
- ➢ Day Blindness
- ➢ Color Blindness
- ➢ Dry Eyes
- ➢ Watering Eyes
- ➢ Iritis
- ➢ Trachoma
- ➢ Squint

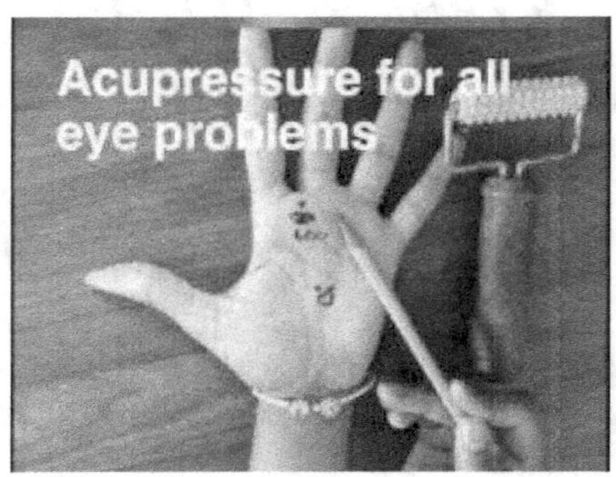

Home Remedies for Eye Problems:

- **Salt water:** Salt water, or saline, is one of the most effective home remedies for eye infections.
- **Tea bags:** Placing cooled tea bags on your eyes while they're closed can be a way to relax and unwind. Some say that it can be an effective home treatment for eye infections.
- **Warm compress:** If your eyes are sore, infected, or irritated, a warm compress can help.
- **Cold compress:** Like warm compresses, cold compresses don't exactly cure eye infections.
- **Wash linens:** Wash your towels and pillow cases daily when you have an eye infection, like conjunctivitis.
- **Discard makeup:** We all know not to share eye makeup, such as mascara, eye shadow, and eye liner, to avoid things like eye infections. But you should also discard your own eye and face makeup, and makeup brushes, while you had an infected eye. This ensures that you won't re-infect yourself.
- **Tips for prevention:** To prevent eye infections, always use the following preventative measures;
- Avoid touching your eyes directly.
- Wash your hands frequently, especially after touching dirty surfaces.
- If you use contact lenses, always clean them and store them correctly.
- Avoid sharing eye makeup or makeup brushes with others.

EAR

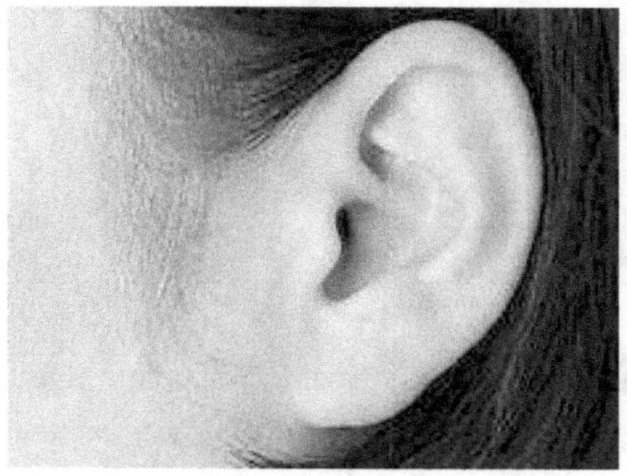

Human Ear: Anatomically, the ear has three distinguishable parts: the outer, middle, and inner ear. The outer ear consists of the visible portion called the auricle, or pinna, which projects from the side of the head, and the short external auditory canal, the inner end of which is closed by the tympanic membrane, commonly called the eardrum.

Common problems of Ear

+ **Ear Infections:** Ear infections are mainly caused by microorganisms like bacteria, fungi, and viruses, and cause symptoms like ear pain, fever, ear blockage, temporary hearing loss, and dizziness.
+ **Hearing Loss:** Hearing loss means total or partial hearing inability in one or both ears. It can be temporary or permanent.
+ **Tinnitus:** Ringing or noise in the ears is known as tinnitus. Inner ear cell damage is the most common cause for this condition.
+ **Meniere's disease:** This is one of the inner ear problems that is characterized by recurring attacks of vertigo, dizziness, nausea, and vomiting. It also causes tinnitus, hearing loss, ear fullness, sweating, and uncontrollable eye movements

Home Remedies for Ear Problems:

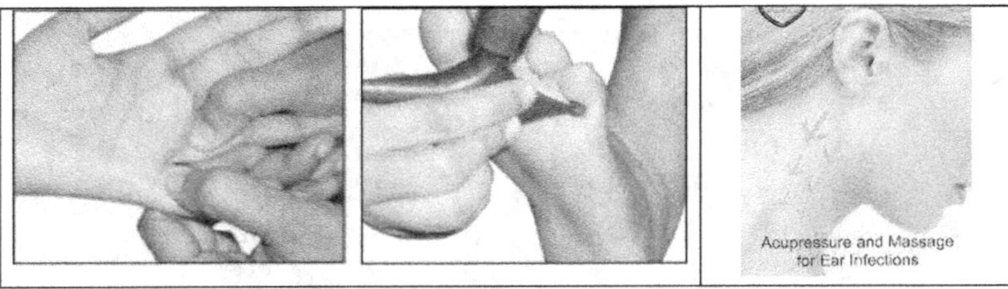

- **A cool or warm compress:** Soak a washcloth in either cool or warm water, wring it out, and then put it over the ear that's bothering you. Try both temperatures to see if one helps you more than the other.
- **A heating pad:** Lay your painful ear on a warm, not hot, heating pad. Over- the-counter ear drops with pain relievers. If they help at all, it's only briefly. You shouldn't use these drops if your eardrum has a tear or hole, so check with your doctor first.
- **Pain reliever:** Acetaminophen, ibuprofen, or naproxen can often relieve the pain of an earache. Ask your doctor which is right for you.
- **Chew gum:** If you're on an airplane or driving at high altitudes and your ear pain is from the change in air pressure, chew some gum. It can help lower that pressure and ease your symptoms.
- **Sleep upright:** While it may sound strange, resting or sleeping sitting up rather than lying down can encourage fluid in your ear to drain. This could ease pressure and pain in your middle ear. Prop yourself up in bed with a stack of pillows, or sleep in an armchair that's a bit reclined.

NOSE

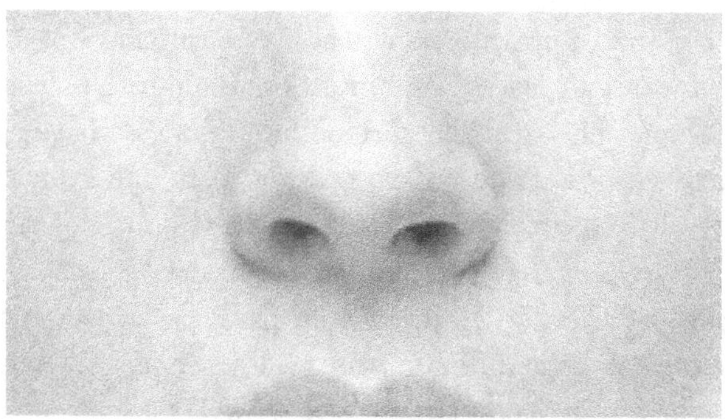

The part of the human face or the forward part of the head of other vertebrates that contains the nostrils and organs of smell and forms the beginning of the respiratory tract.

Common Problems of Nose: Common nose-related issues that ENT's see include; sinus infections, congestion, and airway blockage. Symptoms of sinus infections are pain in your face, upper teeth or in your ear, and drainage that is obstructed or abnormal, or nasal congestion. Symptoms of congestion include feelings of pressure in your head, headaches, and dizziness. Airway blockage of the nose is not being able to breathe properly through the nose.

Reasons for these symptoms can range from allergies, to viral or bacterial infections to a deviated septum. Polyps may also be the culprit in airway blockage.

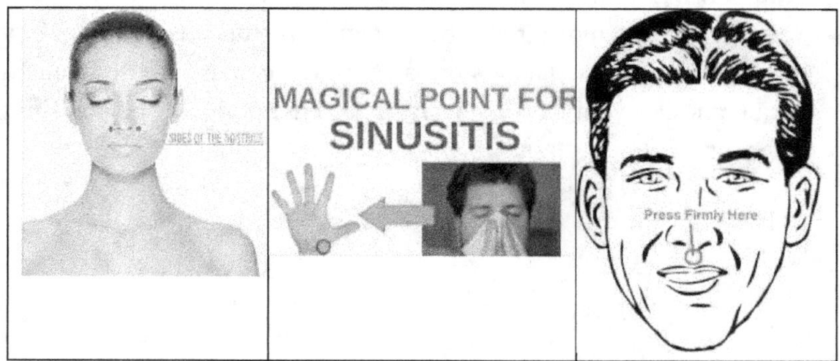

Home Remedies:

- **Flush:** Use a Neti pot, a therapy that uses a salt and water solution, to flush your nasal passages. Nasal irrigation using the Neti pot has been a tried-and- true sinus treatment method for centuries. I have patients who swear by Neti pots and use them daily or weekly to keep their sinuses flowing well. Remember to use distilled water only.

- **Spray**: Use an over-the-counter nasal decongestant spray that contains salt water to help keep your nasal passages moist, unblock congestion and treat inflammation. Some sprays, like Afrin®, can only be used for a maximum of three days. If you exceed three days, you will get "rebound" or worse nasal congestion. Other nasal sprays, like fluticasone, are more effective the longer you use them.

- **Hydrate**: Drink a lot of fluids—water and/or juice—to help thin your mucus. Avoid caffeinated or alcoholic beverages, which can cause dehydration.

- **Rest**: Get plenty of rest to help your body fight infection and speed up recovery. While you sleep, prop yourself up with a couple of pillows. Staying elevated can help you breathe more comfortably.

- **Steam**: Breathe in steam from a pot or bowl of warm (not too hot!) water or take a hot shower. You also can place a warm, wet towel on your face, followed by a cool towel. To help ease sinus pain and open your nasal passages.

- **Spice**: Eat spicy foods to help clear your nasal passages. Add hot peppers, hot sauce, horseradish or wasabi to your meal.

- **Add humidity**: Use a humidifier or vaporizer in your room while you sleep to add moisture to the air and help reduce congestion. Dry air, tobacco smoke and chlorinated water can irritate the mucus membranes in your nose and create an environment ripe for sinus infection.

+ **OTC medication:** Take over-the-counter decongestants, antihistamines (if allergies are the culprit) and pain relievers to reduce sinus pain and pressure. Be sure to check with your doctor first if you have any health issues or take other medicines. Never give decongestants or any over-the-counter cold medicine to children under age 4. Nasal suction is the best form of "decongesting" for young children. This also reduces post-nasal drip and overall lung irritation.
+ **C is key**: Up your intake of vitamin C. This may help fight off sinus infection faster, reduce sinus inflammation and relieve the duration of a sinus infection or cold symptoms.

SOLAR PLEXUS

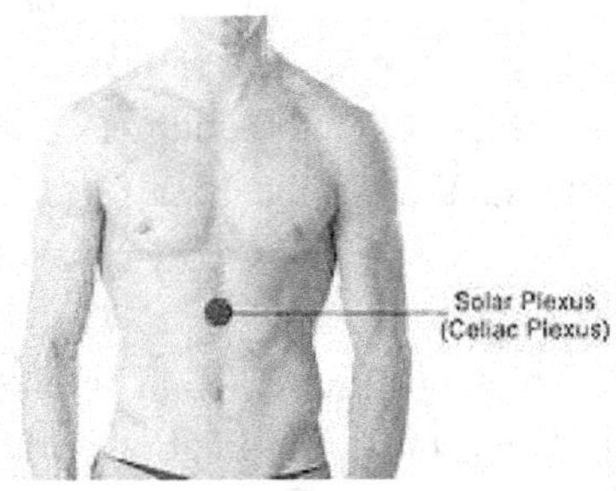

In the human body, a complex collection of nerves of the nervous system in one specific location is known as a „plexus". Thus, the solar plexus is a location where a number of nerve endings meet, which increases the

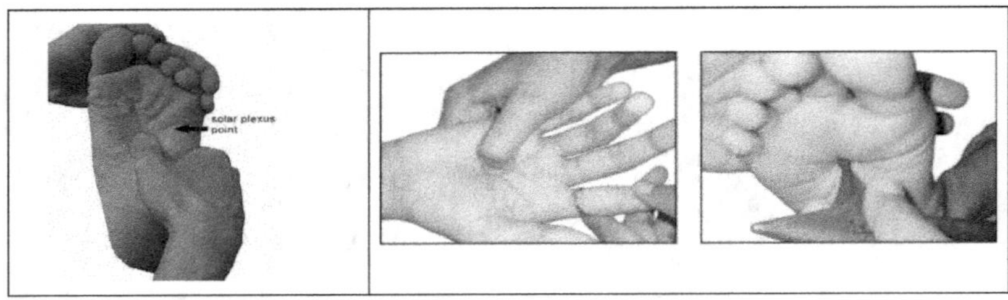

sensitivity and functionality of this specific region.

Home Remedies:

+ **Release any anger you store inside:** When done in conjunction with grounding, releasing pent up anger can help you to unblock your solar plexus quite rapidly. Our congested power is often expressed as blocked anger (just think of the "angry" explosions of volcanoes!), so when we release that anger, we can access that energy again. Try releasing your anger in a healthy way such as through vigorous exercise, punching, kickboxing, dancing, singing, and writing, crying or expressing it through art.

- **Stop seeing yourself as a "victim"**: One of the most damaging mindsets carried by those with blocked solar plexus chakras is the notion that they are "powerless" and defenseless victims of life. If you carry this mentality, it will manifest as the tendency to blame other people for your unhappiness. You might also find yourself constantly sacrificing your needs for others who don't always appreciate your efforts.

- **Repeat the following affirmations:** Reclaim your personal power by repeating the following affirmations: "I can," "I will," "I have the power to decide," "I am strong and courageous," "I embrace my strength," "I love the person I am," "I stand up for myself," "I am responsible for my life," "I am worthy of love and kindness," "I am whole." The more you repeat these affirmations with sincerity, the more they will reprogram your unconscious mind, and therefore, open your solar plexus chakra. Try starting each morning with one of these affirmations.

- **Eat more of these foods**: Eat whole grains such as rice, oats, spelt, and rye which are all great for digestion. Try including more legumes in your diet such as lentils, chickpeas, and beans. Add spices such as turmeric, ginger, cumin, and cinnamon to your food as these spices are heating to the body. Also include yellow fruit and vegetables such as lemons, bananas, corn, pineapple, and yellow capsicums into your eating plan

CERVICAL SPONDYLITIS

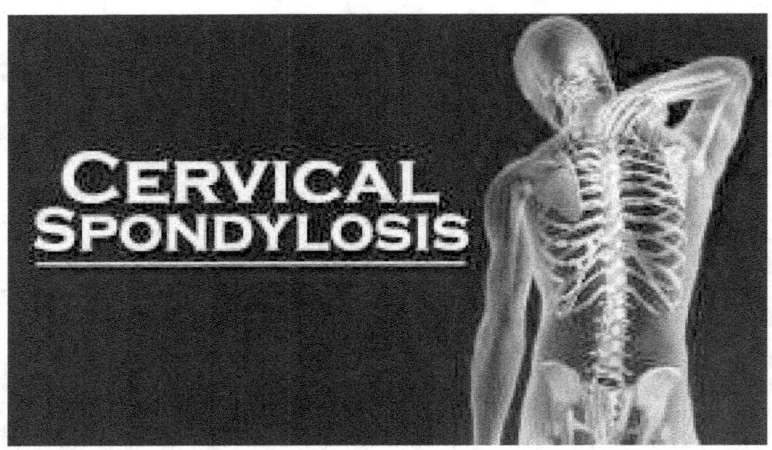

Cervical spondylitis is a general term for age-related wear and tear affecting the spinal disks in your neck. As the disks dehydrate and shrink, signs of osteoarthritis develop, including bony projections along the edges of bones (bone spurs).

Cervical spondylosis is very common and worsens with age. More than 85 percent of people older than age 60 are affected by cervical spondylosis.

Most people experience no symptoms from these problems. When symptoms do occur, nonsurgical treatments often are effective.

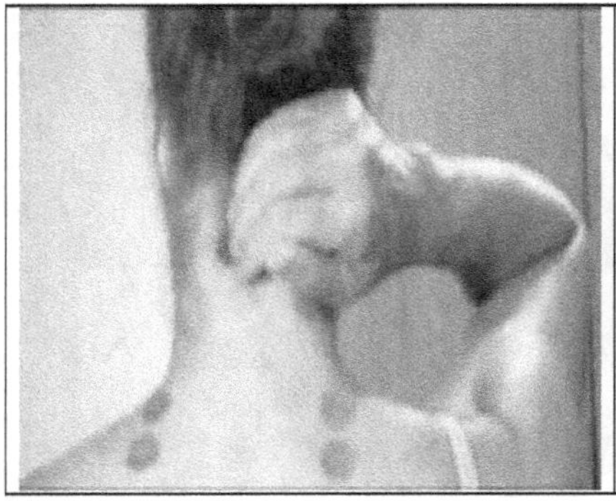
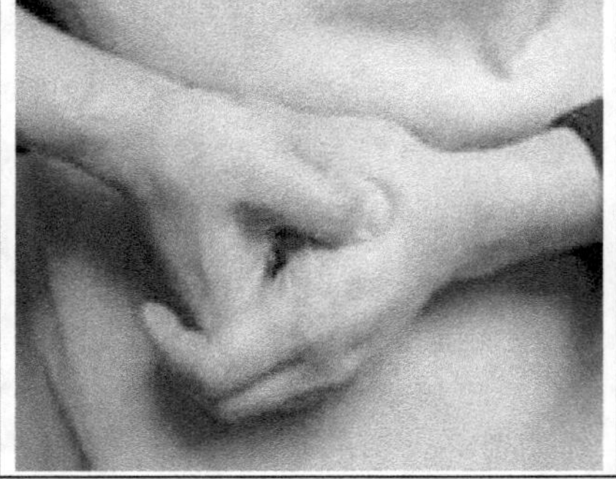

Home Remedies:

- **Regular Exercise**: One of the major causes of cervical spondylosis is lack of regular exercise. Therefore, you can reduce the pain and stiffness around your neck and shoulders by incorporating regular physical exercise into your lifestyle.
- **Cervical Traction**: At times, your doctor may prescribe cervical traction to treat your cervical spondylosis. It is a popular treatment option to deal with neck pain. It is mostly used as part of a physical therapy treatment.
- **Hot and Cold Compresses**: Another easy way to deal with neck pain due to cervical spondylosis is alternating hot and cold compresses on the affected area.
- **Epsom Salt Bath:** Taking an Epsom salt bath on a regular basis is another good remedy to ease the symptoms related to cervical spondylosis. The magnesium in Epsom salt regulates the pH levels in the body, in turn reducing stiffness, inflammation, and pain in the neck and shoulders.
- **Massage**: When it comes to dealing with stiffness or pain in the neck due to cervical spondylosis, massage is a good treatment option.
- **Turmeric**: Due to its anti-inflammatory properties, turmeric is another popular remedy for the pain and inflammation caused by cervical spondylosis. In addition, turmeric increases blood circulation, which helps reduce muscle stiffness and pain.
- **Cayenne Pepper**: Another effective home remedy for finding relief from the pain and inflammation caused by cervical spondylosis is cayenne pepper. It contains capsaicin, which has analgesic as well as anti-inflammatory properties that help reduce pain and inflammation in the neck.
- **Ginger**: Ginger is another widely used home remedy to find relief from the pain and inflammation caused by cervical spondylosis. This herb is rich in anti-inflammatory properties and improves your blood circulation. Thus, it may help reduce pain and inflammation in the neck and surrounding

LOWER BACK PAIN

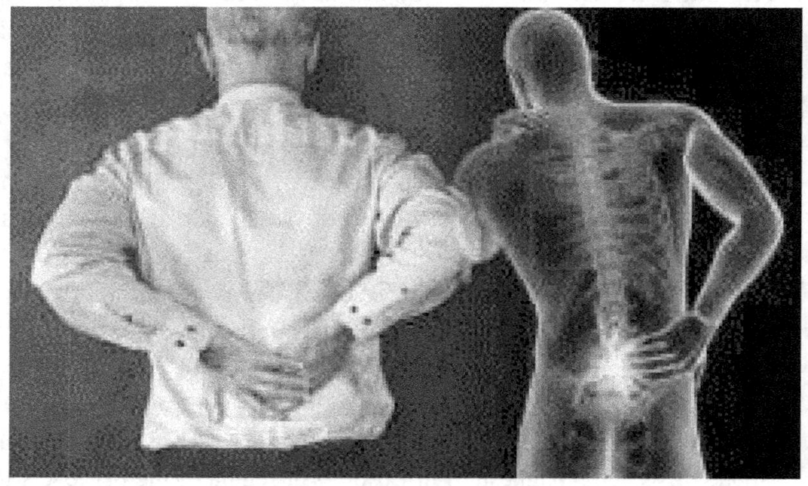

Back pain is one of the most common reasons people go to the doctor or miss work, and it is a leading cause of disability worldwide.

Back pain can range from a muscle aching to a shooting, burning or stabbing sensation. In addition, the pain may radiate down your leg or worsen with bending, twisting, lifting, standing or walking.

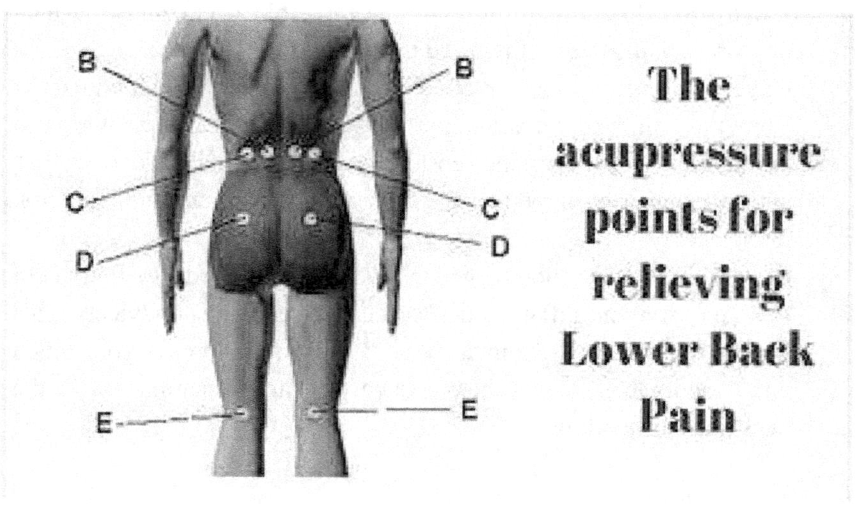

Home Remedies:

✦ **Manage your Stress:** Deep breathing, watching a funny movie, reading a good book, and listening to your favorite music helps.

✦ **Start Eating Healthier**: It is no secret that our diet and the toxins we expose ourselves can be culprits for pain. Start limiting your caffeine intake and eliminate processed and sugary foods. Start eating more lean meats, whole grains and whole foods, and lots of vegetables and greens. Eating more greens will also help balance your pH which is important because when you are stressed you tend to produce more acid creating a disruption in homeostasis.

✦ **Stay Hydrated**: Focus on drinking water and herbal teas. Avoid sugary drinks and lots of caffeine because they can increase inflammation and pain.

✦ **Take a walk:** Walking outside in nature is one of the best exercises you can do. Walking helps you to relax overall as well as gently work your muscles.

✦ Take some Supplements to support structural health. (Use Magnetic Back & Belly Belt).

LOW BLOOD PRESSURE

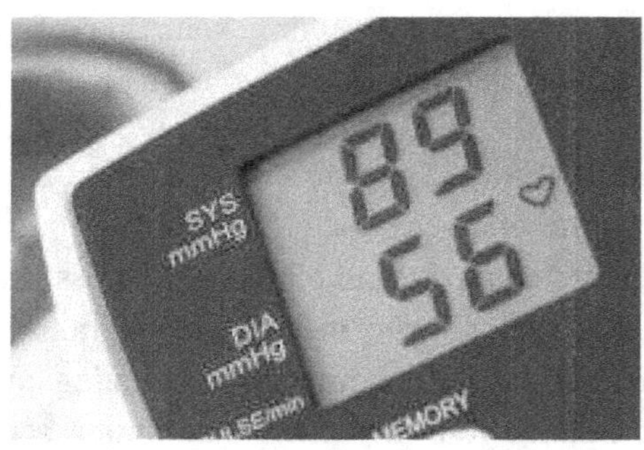

Low blood pressure might seem desirable, and for some people, it causes no problems. However, for many people, abnormally low blood pressure (hypotension) can cause dizziness and fainting. In severe cases, low blood pressure can be life-threatening.

A blood pressure reading lower than 90 millimeters of mercury (mm Hg) for the top number (systolic) or 60 mm Hg for the bottom number (diastolic) is generally considered low blood pressure.

The causes of low blood pressure can range from dehydration to serious medical disorders. It's important to find out what's causing your low blood pressure so that it can be treated.

Apply gentle pressure for 30 seconds 3 times

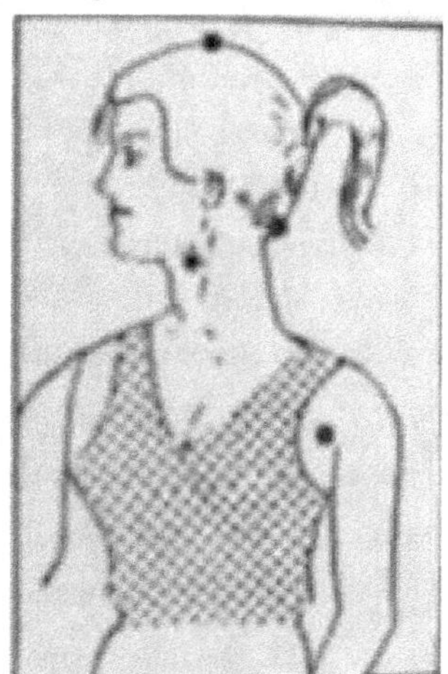

On all points indicated in the above picture

Home Remedies:

- Increase water intake
- Consume more sodium
- Avoid alcohol intake
- Stay active
- Wear compression stockings.
- Avoid staying in heat for long time
- Use extra pillows
- Include caffeine in your diet
- Consume healthy diet
- Consult your doctor

HIGH BLOOD PRESSURE

High blood pressure (HBP or hypertension) is when your blood pressure, the force of your blood pushing against the walls of your blood vessels, is consistently too high.

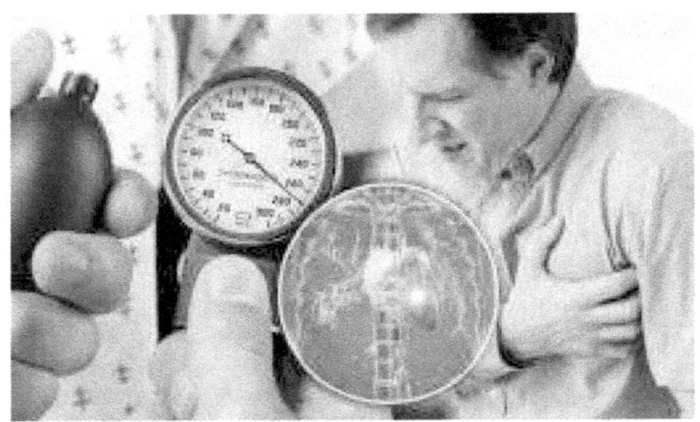

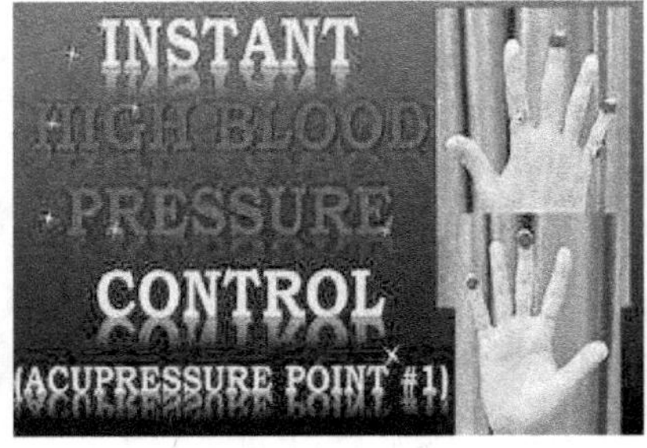

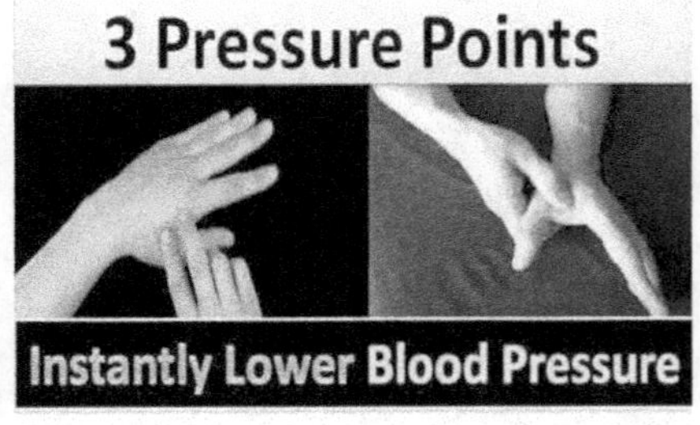

Home Remedies:
- Coconut water
- Celery
- Banana
- Garlic
- Watermelon seeds
- Lemon
- Fenugreek seeds
- Onion Juice
- Cayenne Pepper

HEADACHES

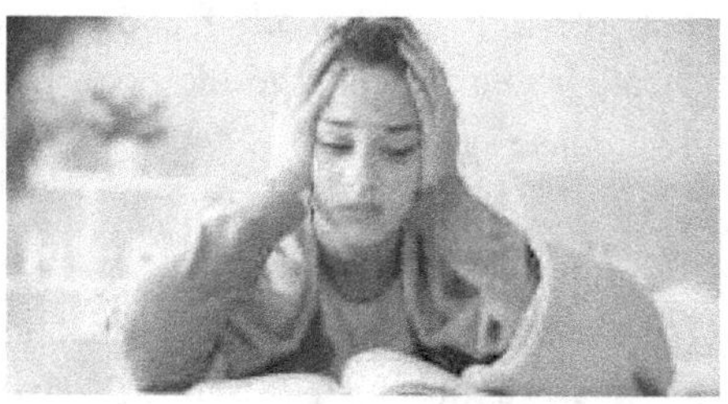

Headaches are a very common condition that most people will experience many times during their lives. The main symptom of a headache is a pain in your head or face. This can be throbbing, constant, sharp or dull.

Home Remedies: -

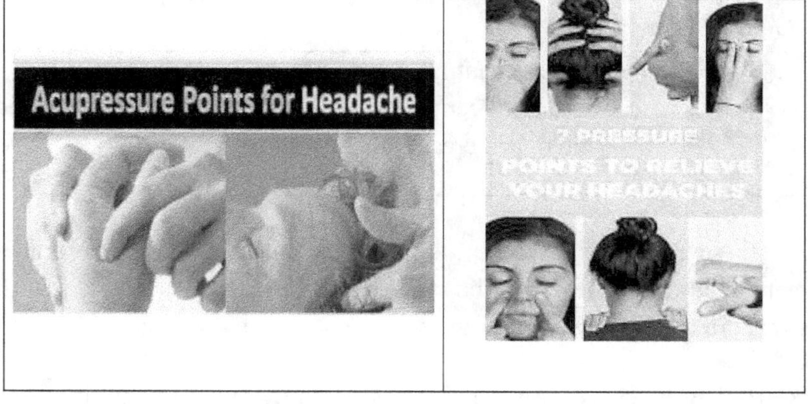

- The best home remedies for headaches include cold or hot compresses, acupressure, and relaxation techniques.
- You should make sure you drink lots of water, improve your diet, and take vitamins or supplements to relieve headache pain.
- Take some sips of ginger tea.
- Use aroma oils for massage.
- Limit screen time.

USEFUL AND IMPORTANT HEALTH TIPS

In order to get speedy recovery, faster relief and to break the vicious cycle of diseases it is advisable to recharge the body battery in order to empower the immune defense system;

23.1.   Copper/Silver/Gold & Iron Charged Water

Copper 50 Grams	Useful for diseases and problems connected with the nervous system such as; High B.P., Arthritis, Polio, Tension and Leprosy.
Silver 20 grams	Useful for the disease of organs connected with digestive and urinary systems.
Gold 10 grams	Useful for disorders of the breathing system, lungs, heart, brain and a General Tonic.
Iron 60 grams	Proper quantity of iron in blood is utmost necessary because it carry Oxygen and supply it all over the body and thus increases Stamina.

All these metals can be put together in water in the proportion as mentioned above. It should be borne in mind that all metals put in the water are thoroughly cleaned and do not contain any dust & rust.

✚ Boil away 25% of water (put 4 glass of water for boiling till it reduces to 3 glasses, filter it and drink it lukewarm during the day.

✚ Drinking one glass of such water first in the morning is very beneficial.

✚ When this water is reduced to 50% it becomes medicine – best antibiotic and is a MUST in treatment of all serious diseases.

+ Avoid sour things like lemon, sour buttermilk etc.

+ The charged water is found useful for good health.

+ But it is a must for the treatment of any problems connected with the improper flow of the current of bio-electricity – High Blood Pressure, Polio, Rheumatism, Arthritis, Paralysis, and Chronic Diseases including Cancer.

+ The use of concentrated Gold water has given wonderful results in the case of mental retardation, muscular dystrophy, T.B., Heart attack etc., and it's a very good brain tonic too.

23.2. Natural Ways to Improve Hemoglobin

+ Eat Iron-Rich Foods Iron deficiency is the most common cause of low Hemoglobin levels.

+ Increase Vitamin C Intake.

+ Increase Folic Acid Intake.

+ You can either eat 1 apple a day, or drink juice made with ½ cup each of apple and beetroot juice twice a day.

+ Avoid eating foods that can block your body's ability to absorb iron, especially if you have a low hemoglobin count i.e., coffee, tea, cola drinks, wine, beer, etc.

+ Exercise

+ Moderate to high intensity workouts are highly recommended, because when you exercise - your body produces more hemoglobin to meet the increasing demand for oxygen throughout the body.
Eating a balanced diet is the best way to ensure you get a daily supply of all essential nutrients...

23.3. People who are struggling with these 3 Health related problems, don't consume ORANGE- can be harmful

The most fruit you see in the market during the cold season is orange. The orange is as beautiful in appearance as it is excellent in taste. These

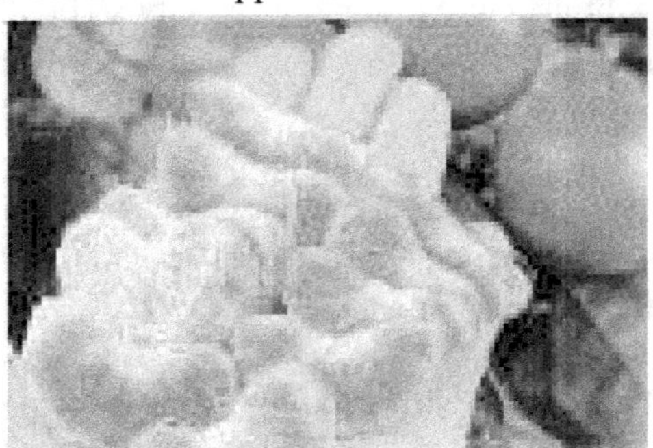

fruits containing vitamin C are also helpful in boosting your immunity. But as you know, excess of anything in the body is harmful for health. In such a situation, if you eat more oranges than necessary, then it also starts negatively affecting your health. Know which people should avoid consuming orange in case of problem related to digestion

If a person has digestive problems, he should avoid orange. This is because oranges are high in fiber. Although fiber is good for health, but if you consume it more than it can increase your stomach problems. It can also cause problems such as cramps, diarrhea and indigestion. Therefore, people struggling with digestion should avoid consuming orange.

If you consume too much of orange, it may affect your teeth. This is because oranges contain acids. This acid combines with calcium present in the enamel of the teeth and can cause bacterial infections. If this happens, there may be cavities in your teeth.

The problem of acidity can increase further if you are struggling with the problem of acidity and consume oranges then it can increase your problem further. Actually, oranges contain acid which can further aggravate this problem. There may even be a burning sensation in your chest and abdomen.

23.4. Risks of Sitting Too Much

Don't let long hours on the sofa wreck your health.

+ **It Hurts Your Heart: -** Scientists first noticed something was up in study that compared two similar groups: transit drivers, who sit most of the day, and conductors or guards who don't. Though their diets and lifestyles were a lot alike, those that sat were about twice as likely to get heart disease as those that stood.

+ **It Can Shorten Your Life: -** You're more likely to die earlier from any cause if you sit for long stretches at a time. It doesn't help if you exercise every day or not. Of course, that's no excuse to skip the gym. If you do that, your time may be even shorter.

+ **Dementia Is More Likely: -** If you sit too much, your brain could look just like that of some with dementia. Sitting also raises your risk of heart disease, diabetes, stroke, high blood pressure, and high cholesterol, which all play a role in the condition. Moving throughout the day can help even more than exercise to lower your risk of all these health problems.

+ **You'll Undo All That Exercise: -** The effects of too much sitting are hard to counter with exercise. Even if you work out 7 hours a week- far more than the suggested 2-3 hours- you can't reverse the effects of sitting 7 hours at a time. Don't throw away all that hard work at gym by hitting the couch for the rest of the day. Keep moving!

+ **Your Odds of Diabetes Rise: -** Yup, you're more likely to have it, too, if you sit all day. And it isn't only because you burn fewer calories. It's the actual sitting that seems to do it. It isn't clear why, but doctors think sitting may change the way your body reacts to insulin, the hormone that helps it burn sugar and carbs for energy.

+ **You Could Get DVT: -** Deep vein thrombosis (DVT) is a clot form in your leg, often because you sit still for too long. It can be serious if the clot breaks free and lodges in your lung. You might notice swelling and pain, but some people have no symptoms. That's why it's a good idea to break up long sitting sessions.

✠ **You'll Gain Weight:-** Watch a lot of TV? Surf the web for hours on end? You're more likely to be overweight or obese. If you exercise every day, that's good, but it won't make a huge dent in extra weight you gain as a result of too much screen time.

✠ **Your Anxiety Might Spike: -** It could be that you're often by yourself and engaged in a screen based activity. If this disrupts your sleep, you can get even more anxious. Plus too much alone time can make you withdraw from friends and loved ones, which is linked to social anxiety. Scientists are still trying to figure out the exact cause.

✠ **It Wrecks Your Back: -** The seated position puts huge stress on your back muscles, neck and spine. It's even worse if you slouch. Look for an ergonomic chair—that means it'll be the right height and support your back in the proper spots. But remember: no matter how comfortable you get, your back still won't like a long sitting sessions. Get up and move around a minute or two every half hour to keep your spine in line.

✠ **It Leads to Varicose Veins: -** Sit for too long and blood can pool in your legs. This puts added pressure in your veins. They could swell, twist or bulge—what doctors call varicose veins. You may also see spider veins, bundles of broken blood vessels nearby. They usually aren't serious, but they can ache. Your doctor can tell you about treatment options if you need them.

✠ **If You Don't Move it, You Could Lose it:-** Older adults who aren't active may more likely to get osteoporosis (weakened bones) and could slowly become unable to perform basic tasks of everyday life, like taking a bath or using the toilet. While moderate exercise won't prevent it. You don't have to go out and run a marathon or take up farming to stay mobile in your golden years. Just don't plant yourself on the couch for hours at a time.

✠ **Your Cancer Risk Goes Up: -** you may be more likely to get colon, endometrial or lung cancer. The more you sit, the higher the odds. Older women have higher odds of breast cancer. That doesn't change if you're super active. What matters is how much you sit.

✚ **How to Take a Stand:-** Work more movements into your day: Stand up and stretch every half hour or so. Touch your toes. Take a stroll around the office. Stand at your desk for part of the day. Get a desk that raises or make your own; Set your computer on top of a box. Talk to your boss about a treadmill desk. All these things can help stop negative effects of uninterrupted sitting and keep you on the road to Good Health.

23.5.   Mistakes That Can Affect Your Cholesterols

Don't skip getting your cholesterol checked-unhealthy numbers typically don't cause symptoms. See how many other no-no's you might be guilty of.

✚ Your Numbers: - Your Cholesterol levels tell your doctor about the fats in your blood. Unhealthy levels are linked to hardening of the arteries which can cause heart disease, heart attacks and strokes. Your numbers include ‒bad‖ (LDL) and ‒good‖ (HDL) cholesterol, and triglycerides, a common fat in your body. If you understand where your numbers are and what may affect them, you can do some things to help manage them

✚ You Don't Get Tested:- Unhealthy cholesterols numbers don't typically cause any symptoms, so it's important to get them checked. If you find out there's a problem, diet, life style changes and medication can help. After 20, your doctor will want to do a simple blood test every 4 to 6 years to make sure they're in healthy range, if your levels are off, your doctor will keep a close eye on them to see if you need treatment.

✚ You Skip Your Workouts: - Regular exercise is one of the best ways to control your cholesterol. You don't have to run a marathon- 40 minutes of walking, swimming, cycling or dancing 3 to 4 times a week will do the trick. If you're short of time, you can break it into 10 minute increments throughout the day. Resistance training- pushups, pull-ups, weights—my help too.

✝ You Park Yourself: - Sitting too long can be linked to obesity, heart disease, and high blood pressure. It lowers –good Cholesterol, which helps get rid of the bad stuff, and raises triglyceride levels. This is true even if you exercise regularly. If you work at desk, try to get up and move around every 30 minutes, or think about using a standing desk.

✝ You Smoke: - It lowers your –good‖ cholesterol levels, which means you, keep more of the bad stuff. And it's linked to high blood pressure, diabetes and heart disease. Quitting can make your cholesterol levels better and help protect your arteries. If you don't smoke, do your best to stay away from second hand smoke.

✝ You Ignore Your Weight: - Carrying too many pounds, especially around your belly, can raise bad cholesterol (LDL) and Lower good kind (HDL). But loose just 10% of your weight and you could really help your numbers. Talk to your doctor about the best diet and exercise program to help you lose weight.

✝ You Eat a Lot of Saturated Fat: - This comes from beef, pork, lamb and full fat dairy like butter, cream, milk, cheese and yoghurt as well as tropical oils like palm and coconut. All those things can rise your LDL, or –bad Cholesterol. It can help to trim visible fat from meats and go with skim milk and low fat yoghurt. If your LDL is high, you shouldn't get than 6% of your calories from the saturated fat.

✝ You Eat a Lot of Trans Fat: - Sometimes called —partially hydrogenated —fats or oils, you find them in fried foods, pastries, pizza dough, doughnuts, muffins, cookies, crackers, and many prepackaged foods. They raise your bad cholesterol levels and lower the good stuff, Check food labels to limit trans fats, eat plenty of fruits, vegetables, whole grain, low fat dairy, poultry, fish and nuts.

✝ You cut Out all Fats:- They're not all bad. Replace saturated and Trans fats with healthier polyunsaturated and monounsaturated fats. You'll find those fats in trout, salmon, herring, avocados, olives, walnuts and lipid vegetable oil like sunflower, canola, and olive oil. But make sure no more than 30% of your daily calories come from any kind of fat.

✝ You Forget About Fiber:- These are 2 types; soluble, which dissolves in water and insoluble, which doesn't. Both are good for your heart health. But soluble fiber in particular helps lower your LDL levels. Add it to your diet with a bowl of oatmeal in the morning or with oat bran, fruits, beans, lentils or vegetables.

+ You Drink Too Much: - overdoing it with alcohol can cause unhealthy cholesterol numbers. In particular, it can raise the level of fats in your blood. Men should have no more than two drinks per day, and women one. If you keep that, you also might boost your HDL or good cholesterol numbers.

+ You ignore other Conditions: - It's important to understand and treat any medical issues linked to bad cholesterol numbers like high blood pressure, diabetes, kidney disease, liver disease and hypothyroidism. If you have one of those conditions and manage it well, you may help your numbers, too. You Skip Your Medication Sometimes: - Follow your doctor's directions about any prescriptions. If you do forget to take your medicine, don't try to —make up‖ doses by taking more the next time. It may not work the way it's supposed to, or it may make you dizzy or sick. Make sure to tell your doctor about any drug you already take. Some drugs can cause problems if they're taken at the same time as other meds.

23.6.   For Healthier Eyes

A few smart moves can protect your eyes from the wear and tear of daily life. Here's what you should be doing.

+ **Take a 20 second Computer Break: -** Staring at a computer (or any digital screen) won't hurt your eyes, but it can make them feel tired and dry. Surprisingly, we blink about half as often when we're looking at the screen. Follow the 20/20/20 rule: Every 20 minute, look at least 20 feet away for at least 20 seconds. Also place your screen so it's about 25 inches away and slightly below eye level. Cut glare by moving light sources or using a screen filter.

+ **Always Wear Sunglasses: -** UV radiation can hurt your eyes just like it does your skin. Effects add up and can cause problems like cataracts, cornea burns, and even cancer of eyelid. Whenever you're outside-even on cloudy days – wear sunglasses or contacts that block 99% to 100% of UV-A and UV –B rays. Protective lenses don't have to be expensive, just check the label. Hats block exposure, too. Snow, water, sand and concrete all can reflect UV rays.

Use Safety Glasses at Work and Play: - Nearly half of eye injuries happen at home, not on a job site. Use safety glasses whenever a project might send debris flying or splash hazardous chemicals. Protective eyewear may prevent 90% of sports – related eye injuries. Lenses should be made of poly carbonated plastic – which is 10 times more impact resistant than other materials. Some sports with the most injuries are baseball/softball, racket sports, lacrosse and basketball.

Eat for Your Heart and for Your Eyes: - Foods that help circulation are good for your heart, eyes and vision. Choose heart-healthy foods like citrus fruits, dark leafy greens, and whole grains. Foods rich in zinc-beans, peas, peanuts, oysters, lean red meat and poultry – can help eyes resist light damage. And carrots do help eyesight. The Vitamin A in them is important for good vision. Other nutrients that help eyes include beta- carotene (found in many yellow or orange fruits and veggies), and lutein and Zeaxanthin (found in leafy greens and colorful produce)

Don't Ignore Eye Problems: - if your eyes are itchy or red, soothe them with cold compresses antihistamines, or eye drops. If you feel grittiness, like there's sand in your eyes, rinse with clean water or saline. See a doctor if symptoms continue, or if you have pain, secretion, swelling, or sensitivity to light, other reasons to see a doctor: dark floating spots, flashes of light, or any time you can't see normally.

Clean you're Contact Lenses: - Take care of your eyes by taking care of your contacts. Always wash your hands before handling lenses. Use only cleaners and drops approved by your eye doctor clean, rinse and dry the case each time you remove the lenses, and replace it every two to three months. Don't wear when you're swimming or using cleaning products like bleach. Don't leave daily wear lenses in while you sleep, even for a nap. And don't wear lenses longer than the time recommended.

- **Know Your Health History:** - Many seemingly unrelated health conditions can affect your eyes. High blood pressure and diabetes can reduce blood flow to the eyes. Immune system disorders in the lungs, thyroid glands or elsewhere can inflame eyes too, other threats include multiple sclerosis, aneurysms and cancer. Tell your eye doctor about any current or past health issues including family members with the eye problems or serious illnesses.

- **Read Drug Labels:** - Many types of drugs, or combinations of drugs can affect your vision. Be on the lookout for possible side effects from various medications used to treat different conditions. Tell your doctor if you notice issue like dry or watery eyes, double vision, light sensitivity, puffy or droopy eyelids, and blurred vision.

- **Throw Away Old Eye Makeup:** - Bacteria grow easily in liquid or creamy eye makeup. Throw out products after 3 months. If you develop an infection, immediately get rid of all you eye makeup and see a doctor. If you tend to have allergic reactions, try only one new product at a time. Never share cosmetics and don't use store samples. Clean you face thoroughly before and after using makeup, and don't apply cosmetics inside lash lines.

- **Get Regular Eye Exams:** - You should get your eyes checked regularly, even if you don't wear glasses. Ask your doctor how often. It will be at least every year from ages 18-60 or every year if you're older, wear contact lenses or have risk factors like diabetes, high blood pressure, or a family history of eye diseases.

- **Stop Smoking:** - If you smoke, stop. Smoking means dramatic increase in incidence of macular degeneration as well as raising you risk of developing cataracts and aggravating uncomfortable dry eyes. It also builds up plaque in your blood stream and weakens arteries. This not only raise the risk of a heart attack, but it can damage the retina and cause vision loss. The good news is that after you quit, your risk of eye disease is about the same as for non-smokers.

WELLNESS QUOTES

- High stress, high fat intake, high life and high protein foods all contribute to our "un wellness."

- When you get up in the morning and stumble into the bathroom – you can do a simple test by using a little strip of pH paper and a small sample of your urine – you will find either the color changes dramatically, becoming very dark. Or the paper will not change the color only appear to be wet.

- The color of paper is your key to beginning to understand just how healthy you are. If the pH paper turned very dark;

    - You are not healthy even if you feel good and

    - You must not engage in strenuous exercise.

- If the pH paper didn't change the color at all;

    - You are headed to for serious disease if you continue this way.

    - You can still exercise.

- The primary personal responsibility of each of us is to promote our own health, not merely fight disease.

- Medicine's principal objective is to relieve pain and suffering – to make people more comfortable.

- Medicines can't heal; drugs can't heal only the body's strong immune system heals.

- If you're daily diet includes more protein than the equivalent of two eggs and a hamburger, your health is going downhill fast.

- You have a chance and a choice to be as healthy as you decide to be – really you have the ability to help yourself feel better and healthy.

- Your body doesn't know how to be sick; it knows exactly what to do to survive as long as possible.

- Symptoms are the signals that body is adapting its functions to survive the things we do to it. Your body doesn't know how to be sick.

- The food that fuels your body this year dictates how healthy you will be in coming years.
- Anyone who is committed to taking responsibility for his/her own health can reach any level of wellness he/she wants.
- Your actions and reactions determine how healthy you are.
- Feeling good is a wonderful way to live, when you are healthy you not only feel good but you can enjoy life.
- Your body is alkaline by design and acid by function.
- Acid must be either neutralized or eliminated.
- Too much acid is termed acidosis- ACIDOSIS = TOXICITY!
- Always remember that too much protein can lead to toxicity.
- Emotional stress in the form of negative thoughts can have painful consequences.
- Stress producing Thoughts are the most potent toxin producers in your body – Foods are in second place.
- Everyday foods like bread, cereal, fish, chicken and meat affect the acid level of your body, and the acid level of your body affects your health.
- The greatest threat to alkaline reserve is excess protein.
- Food selection and tastes are major elements of lifestyle – Lifestyle can be improved.
- Once you've started to break out in health, the first thing in your stomach should be fruit. It makes no difference if your first meal is at 5am or 2pm – fruit first.
- Quick changes in attitudes and perceptions may causes you distress. Your actions are based on your belief. Your beliefs are based on your past experiences.
- Happiness is part of who we are. Joy is the feeling.
- When health is absent, wisdom cannot reveal itself, art cannot manifest, strength cannot fight, wealth becomes useless, and intelligence cannot be applied.

- "To ensure good health: eat lightly, breathe deeply, live moderately, cultivate cheerfulness, and maintain an interest in life." – William Londen
- "Health is a state of complete mental, social and physical well-being, not merely the absence of disease or infirmity." – World Health Organization, 1948.
- "Focus on health, energy, vitality – not weight." – Karen Salman Sohn
- "The best six doctors anywhere and no one can deny it are sunshine, water, rest, air, exercise and diet."- Wayne Fields
- "Health is a large word. It embraces not the body only, but the mind and spirit as well…and not today's pain or pleasure alone, but the whole being and outlook of a man." – James H. West
- Sleep is that golden chain that ties health and our bodies together.
- Early to bed and early to rise, makes a man healthy wealthy and wise" ~Benjamin Franklin
- "Physical fitness is not only one of the most important keys to a healthy body, it is the basis of dynamic and creative intellectual activity." ~John F. Kennedy
- "The greatest wealth is Health." ~Unknown
- "Let food be thy medicine and medicine be thy food "~Hippocrates
- "Just because you're not sick doesn't mean you're healthy" ~Author Unknown
- "Those who think they have no time for exercise will sooner or later have to find time for illness." ~Edward Stanley

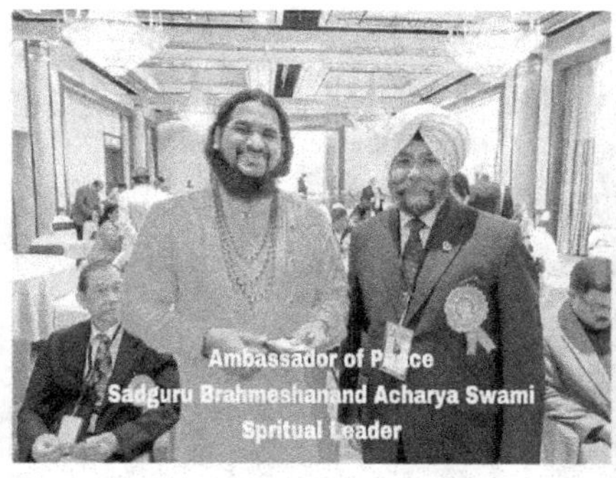
Ambassador of Peace
Sadguru Brahmeshanand Acharya Swami
Spritual Leader

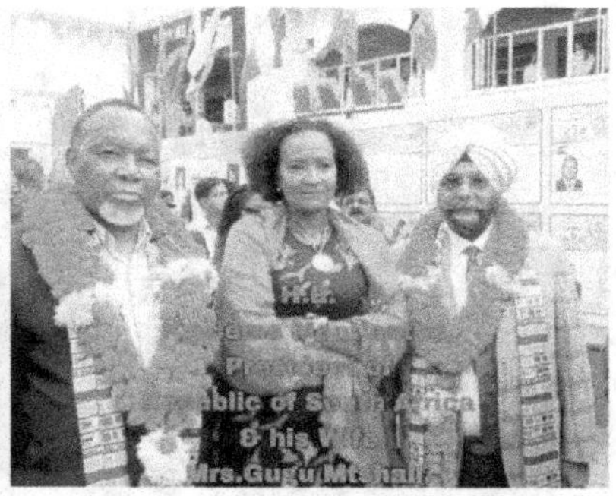

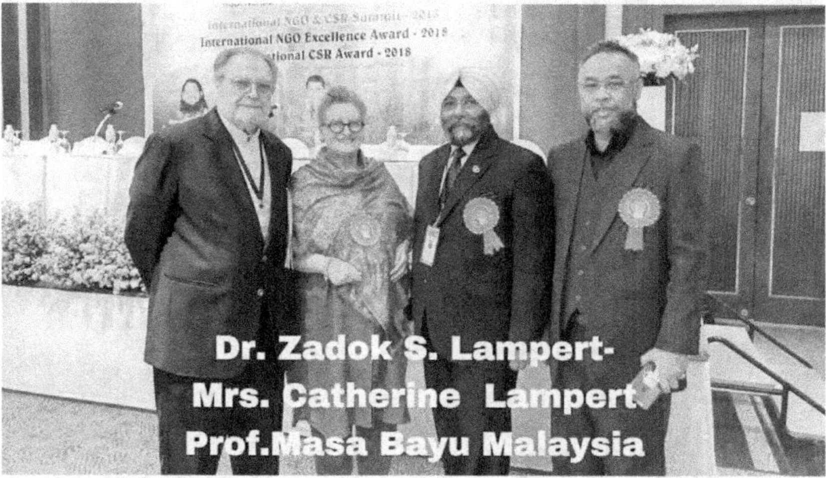
International NGO & CSR Summit - 2018
International NGO Excellence Award - 2018
...tional CSR Award - 2018
Dr. Zadok S. Lampert-
Mrs. Catherine Lampert
Prof.Masa Bayu Malaysia

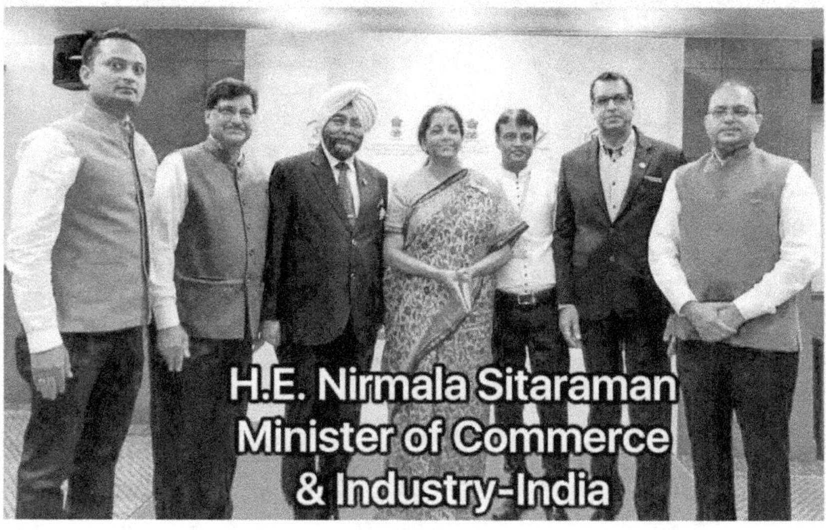
H.E. Nirmala Sitaraman
Minister of Commerce
& Industry-India

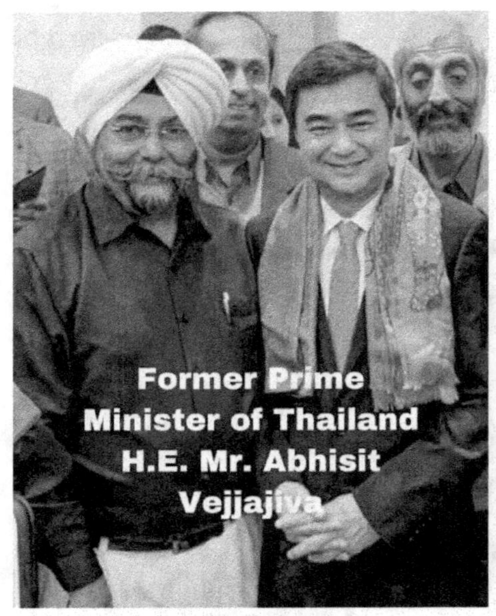

Former Prime
Minister of Thailand
H.E. Mr. Abhisit
Vejjajiva

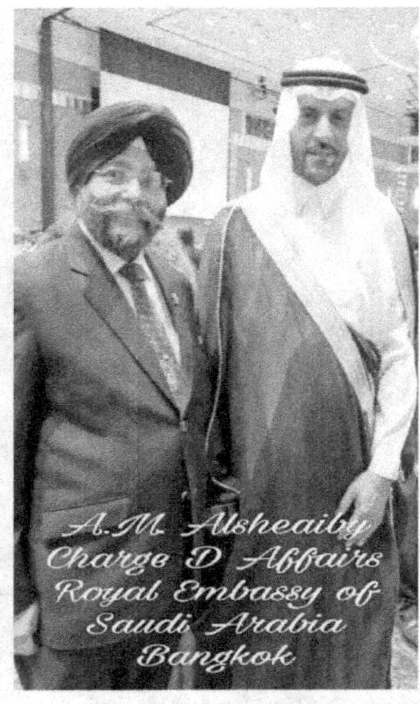

A.M. Alsheaiby
Charge D Affairs
Royal Embassy of
Saudi Arabia
Bangkok

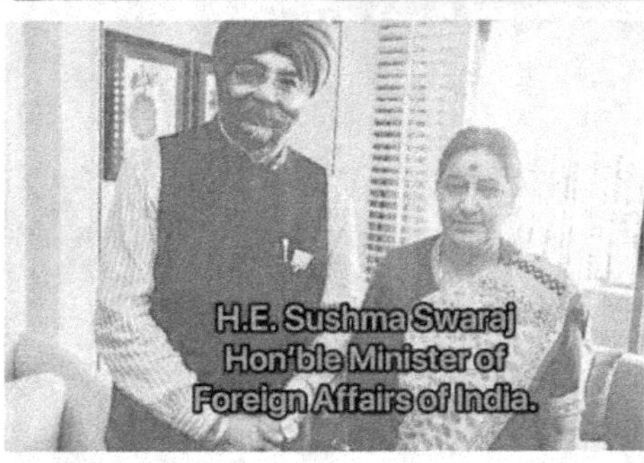

H.E. Sushma Swaraj
Hon'ble Minister of
Foreign Affairs of India.

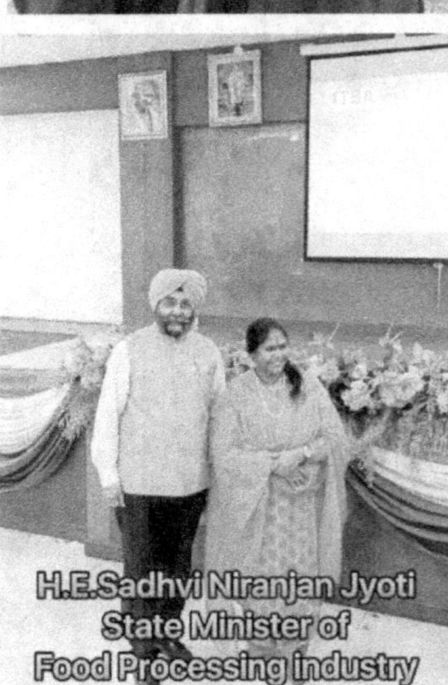

H.E.Sadhvi Niranjan Jyoti
State Minister of
Food Processing industry
of India.

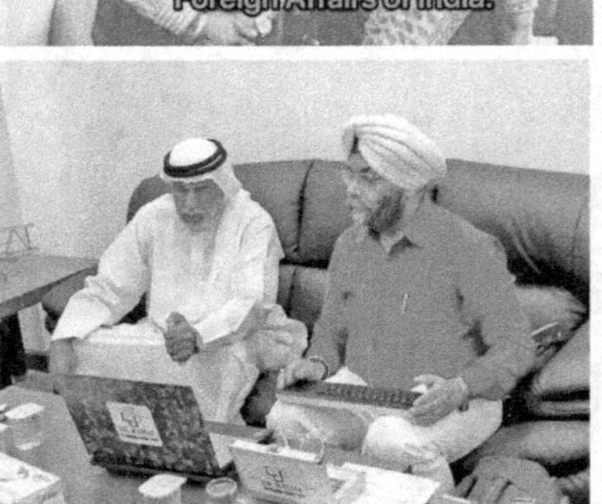

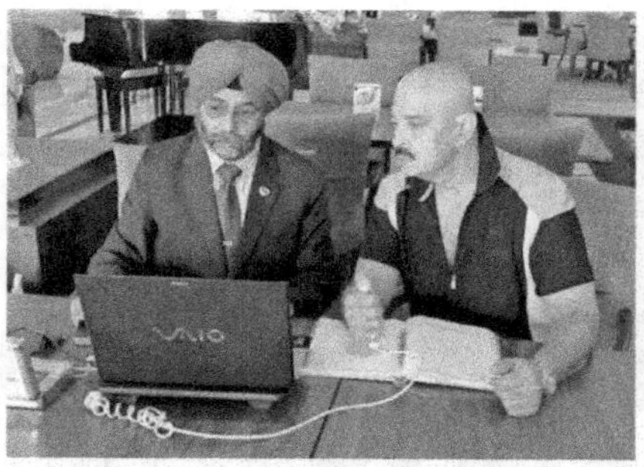

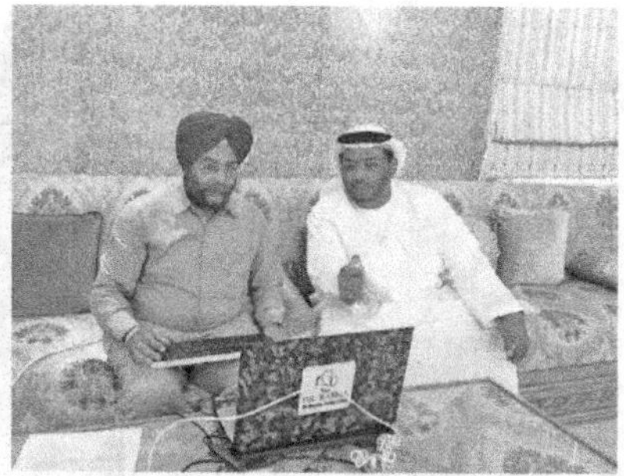

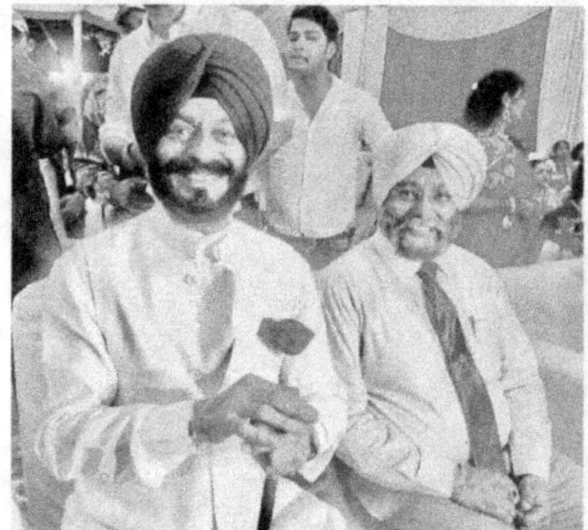

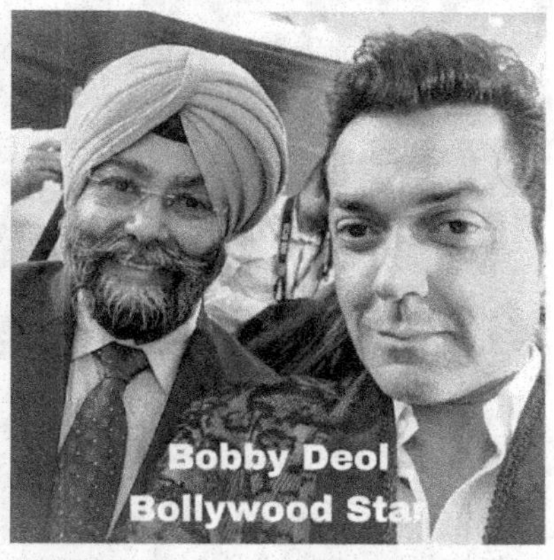
Bobby Deol
Bollywood Star

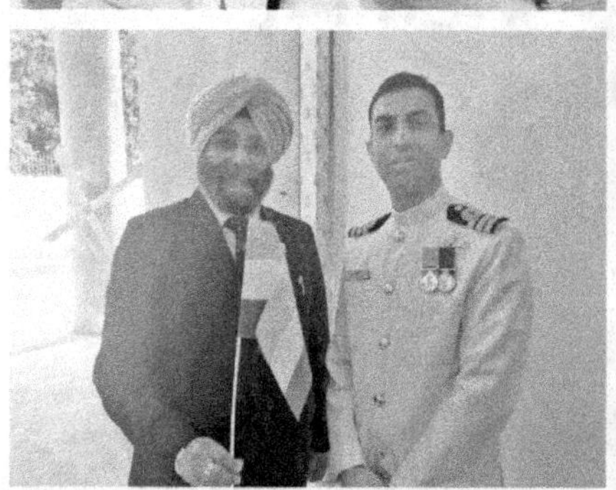

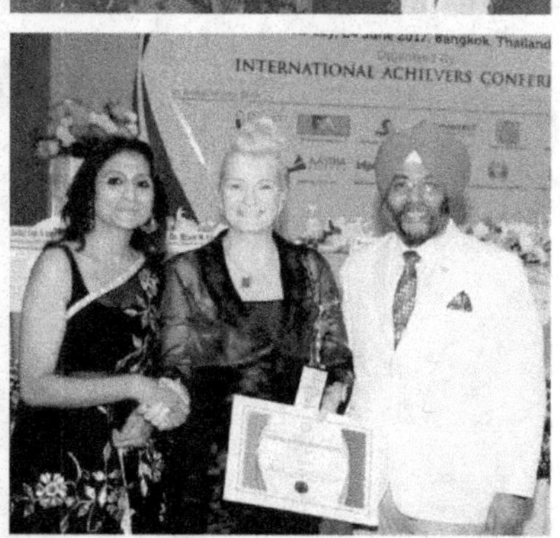
Bangkok, Thailand
INTERNATIONAL ACHIEVERS CONFERE

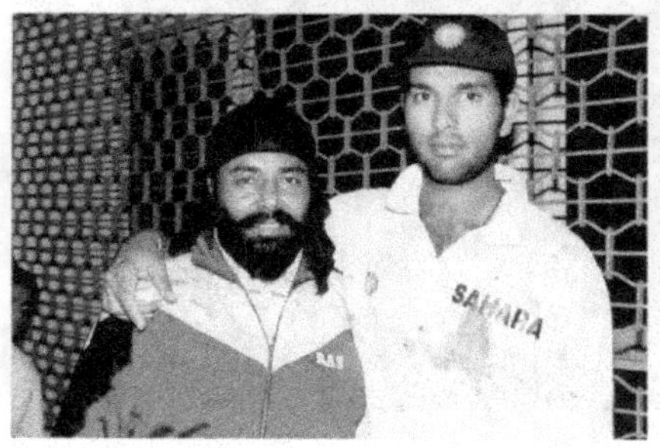

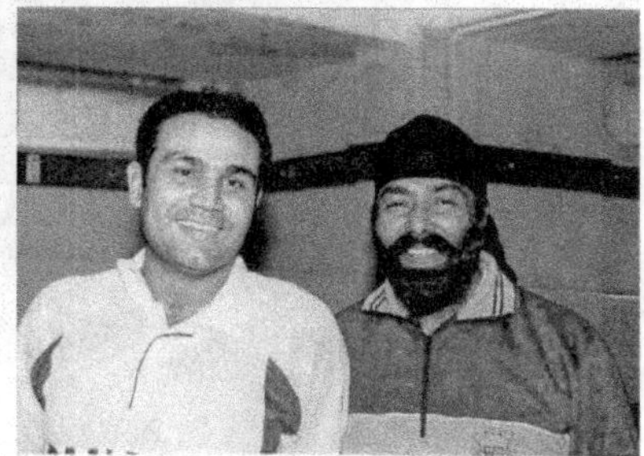

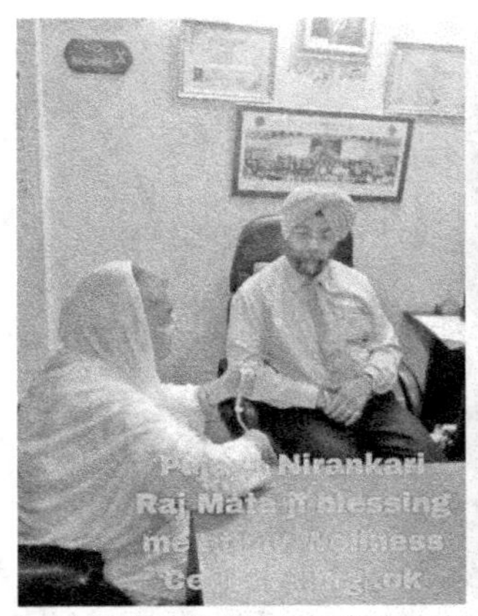
Nirankari
Raj Mata ji blessing
His Holiness

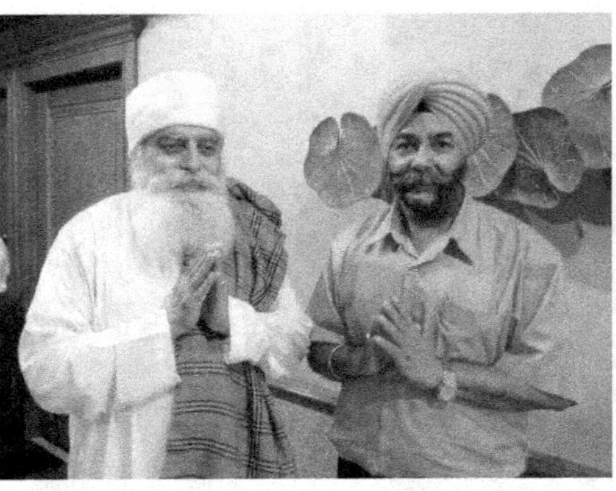

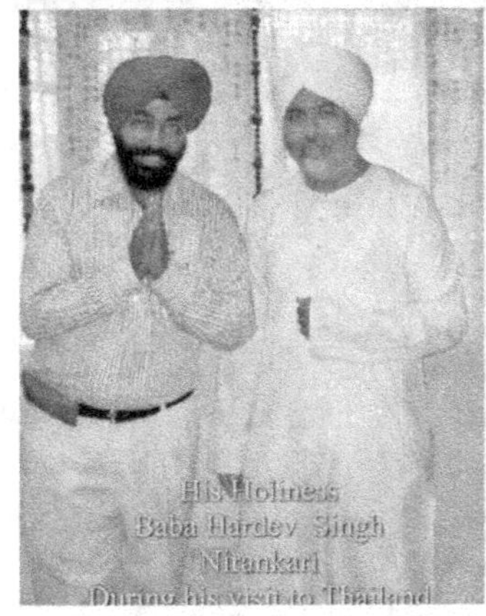
His Holiness
Baba Hardev Singh
Nirankari
During his visit to Thailand

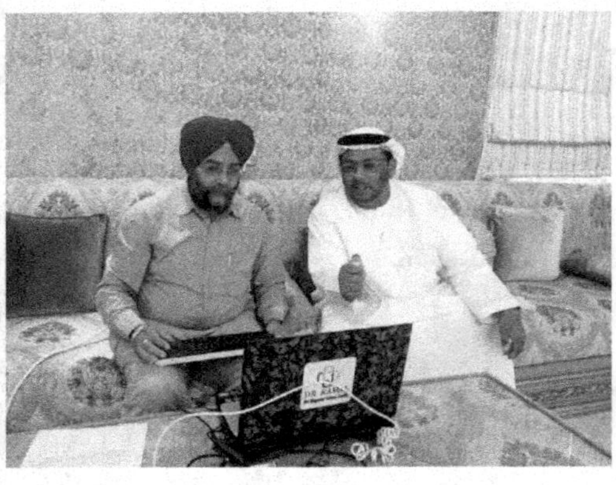

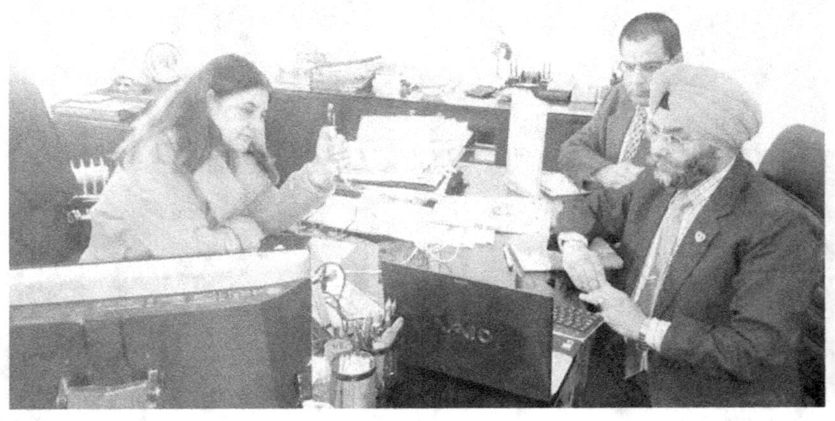

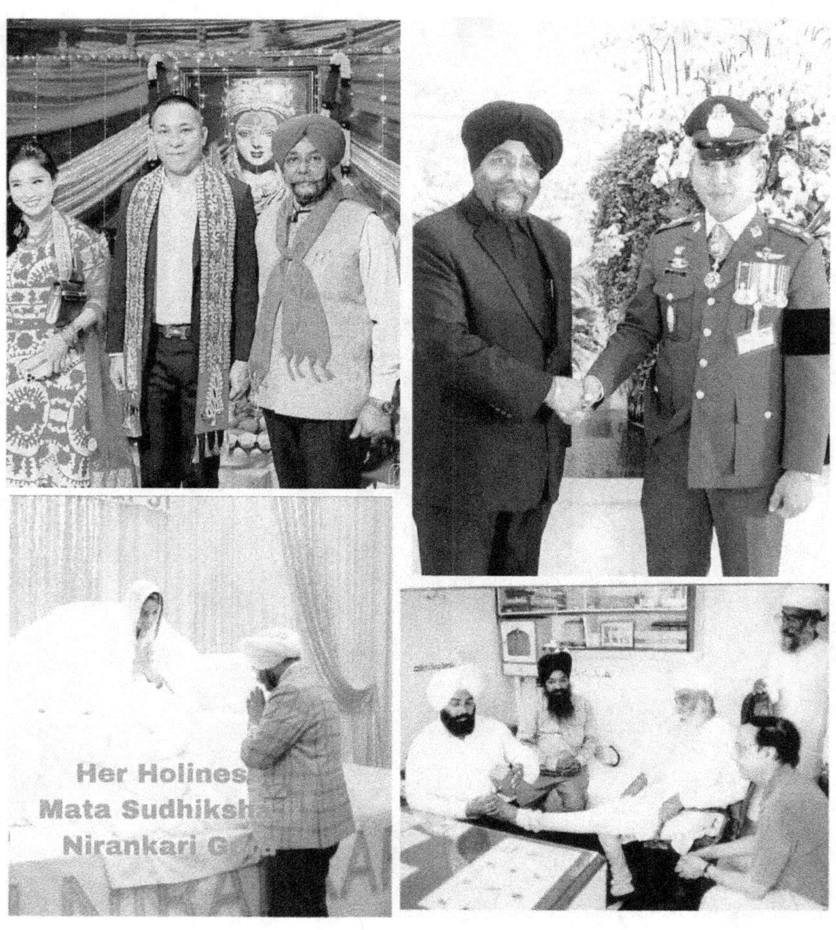
Her Holiness
Mata Sudhiksh
Nirankari G

www.ingramcontent.com/pod-product-compliance
Lightning Source LLC
Chambersburg PA
CBHW071950150726

47999CB00001B/376